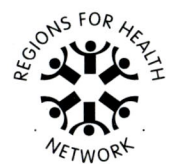 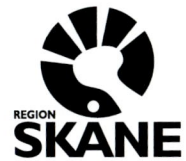 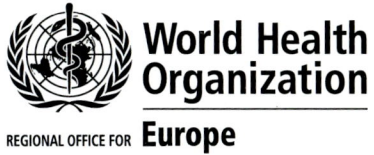

Taking a participatory approach to development and better health

Examples from the Regions for Health Network

Abstract

If the ultimate goal of all development is to improve the prerequisites for long-term survival and the well-being of the population in a region, then this entails action for increased social inclusion and a more equitable distribution of the social determinants of health. The intentional consequences of participatory approaches go far beyond the health sector and more into the realm of creating positive sustainable social change. Through the engagement of stakeholders, recognizing the value of each person's contribution to the process is not only practical but also collaborative and empowering in finding solutions together. WHO's Health 2020 policy calls for a whole-of-government and whole-of-society approach that involves a range of stakeholders at all levels. This publication documents the experiences of participatory approaches taken by Region Skåne (Sweden) and three case studies: the Autonomous Province of Trento (Italy), the Autonomous Community of Andalusia (Spain) and Wales (United Kingdom).

Keywords

CASE STUDIES
HEALTH PLAN IMPLEMENTATION
HEALTH POLICY
PUBLIC HEALTH

Address requests about publications of the WHO Regional Office for Europe to:
    Publications
    WHO Regional Office for Europe
    UN City, Marmorvej 51
    DK-2100 Copenhagen Ø, Denmark
Alternatively, complete an online request form for documentation, health information, or for permission to quote or translate, on the Regional Office web site (http://www.euro.who.int/pubrequest).

ISBN 978 92 890 5112 5
© World Health Organization 2015

All rights reserved. The Regional Office for Europe of the World Health Organization welcomes requests for permission to reproduce or translate its publications, in part or in full.

The designations employed and the presentation of the material in this publication do not imply the expression of any opinion whatsoever on the part of the World Health Organization concerning the legal status of any country, territory, city or area or of its authorities, or concerning the delimitation of its frontiers or boundaries. Dotted lines on maps represent approximate border lines for which there may not yet be full agreement.

The mention of specific companies or of certain manufacturers' products does not imply that they are endorsed or recommended by the World Health Organization in preference to others of a similar nature that are not mentioned. Errors and omissions excepted, the names of proprietary products are distinguished by initial capital letters.

All reasonable precautions have been taken by the World Health Organization to verify the information contained in this publication. However, the published material is being distributed without warranty of any kind, either express or implied. The responsibility for the interpretation and use of the material lies with the reader. In no event shall the World Health Organization be liable for damages arising from its use. The views expressed by authors, editors, or expert groups do not necessarily represent the decisions or the stated policy of the World Health Organization.

Edited by Nancy Gravesen
Book design by Marta Pasqualato
Printed in Italy by AREAGRAPHICA SNC DI TREVISAN GIANCARLO & FIGLI
Cover: © Region Skåne/Anders Tukler

CONTENTS

Foreword .... *v*

Foreword .... *vii*

Acknowledgments ix

Executive summary xi

Background 1

    Implementation of whole-of-government and
whole-of-society approaches 1

    A theoretical framework 3

Setting the scene 9

    Key facts about Skåne 9

    Region Skåne 9

    Skåne's agenda 11

Open Skåne 2030: the process 14

    Internal process 14

    External process 18

    Review period 21

    Adoption 23

Implementation – moving from what to how 24

    Public health 25

    Evaluation 30

Challenges and strengths of the process 33
Challenges 33
Strengths 34
Joint action for development 36
Key messages 38

Case studies 40
Autonomous Province of Trento (Italy) 40
Autonomous Community of Andalusia (Spain) 44
Wales (United Kingdom) 47

References 52

Foreword

What is participation and why does it matter? Participation is one of those all-encompassing concepts of fundamental relevance to any sphere of life: in our personal life, at work and within society. Nothing can be achieved without participation. People who surround us are not only necessary to achieve societal goals, but also crucial for us to achieve our personal goals. Granted that, however, doing things together is all but simple.

Health and well-being are dimensions of life, which result from a complex interplay of different sectors, at different levels, and in all groups of society. When we, at the WHO Regional Office for Europe, encounter so-called champions in a specific field of public health, we feel compelled to document their work as best practice and to share their experience with all our Member States. This is exemplified by Skåne (Sweden) with the regional development strategy described in great depth and by three case studies: in the Autonomous Province of Trento (Italy) with the development of a regional health plan, in the Autonomous Community of Andalusia (Spain) with the Fourth Andalusian Health Plan; and in Wales (United Kingdom) with the Well-being of Future Generations Act 2015.

These case studies stand out for how participation concepts were put at the core of health plans and legislation, and emphasize four elements.

Firstly, participation is a key element in achieving both the whole-of-government and the whole-of-society approaches suggested in Health 2020. Participation is the tool through which both approaches are made possible, in terms of collaboration across various sectors and in vertical coherence among different levels of governance, and in the full involvement of civil societies towards any decision, which can affect their health and well-being.

Secondly, participation is a tool to better understanding. Participatory approaches require the genuine will to understand others and to constructively engage in an enriching dialogue. These case studies describe the inclusive engagement with other sectors and all groups of society, finding in the communities themselves the best possible leverages to increase their social capital.

Thirdly, these plans and legislation are forward-thinking in nature and aim at increasing populations' health and well-being, embedding social equity as a core value and as an instrumental step for sustainable development.

Fourthly, participation is a fundamental element to grant solidity to the policy-making process. Changes in governments can hamper or slow down the policy-making process itself or the implementation of previously adopted policies. However, if these are the results of wide consultations, which listen to the voices of all groups in society, turnover of top officials can indeed bring new nuances to the process and contents, but never alter their essence.

All of this and much more is presented in this publication, which indeed enriches the growing repository of successful experiences around Health 2020 implementation at all levels of governance.

Special thanks go to Region Skåne: first for being at the forefront of participatory approaches prompting better health for all, and secondly for their determination and availability to share what it learnt with the international community.

Piroska Ostlin
Acting Director, Division of Policy and Governance for Health and Well-being
WHO Regional Office for Europe

Foreword

Skåne, Sweden has in many ways aligned its recent development successfully with the demands of the global economy. This has invoked a very visible increase in the exchange of goods, capital and people across its border. This has stimulated success in many important development areas, but the downside of this development might also have become more rapidly visible than in other areas of Sweden. A major challenge for any society in a state of rapid transition is to maintain social sustainability, one of the cornerstones to a continued positive development of population health, particularly improved health equity, and of long-term economic and environmental sustainability.

Skåne today is both multifaceted and contradictory. *It has the highest unemployment level in Sweden, but also strong growth in employment. Never have so many people in Skåne been employed as now. Skåne has a large percentage of highly educated residents, but also an increasing percentage of students who finish compulsory school with very poor results. These paradoxes reflect our current position, here and now.*

The open Skåne 2030 *is the regional development strategy created by Region Skåne, the public organization responsible for health care in Skåne. The strategy is the result of extensive dialogues with citizens, civil society, business and the public sector who are now working together to meet a joint strategic objective: to achieve an open Skåne by 2030 that welcomes pluralism, more people and new ideas; is characterized by high tolerance and widespread participation in common social issues; encompasses an open landscape, as well as urbanization; and offers everyone the chance of a good life.*

In order to attain this vision, five prioritized statements were selected to achieve a completely open Skåne: Skåne shall offer optimism and quality of life; be a strong, sustainable growth engine; benefit from its polycentric urban structure; develop the welfare services of tomorrow; and be globally attractive. This strategy is about how to boost the positive sides of the current development, as well as to reduce its negative effects on social sustainability and population health.

I am also fortunate in this publication to share learning from other members of the WHO Regions for Health Network about participatory approaches, namely the Autonomous Province of Trento (Italy) and the development of a health plan; the Autonomous Community of Andalusia (Spain) and the experience of designing, implementing and assessing the Fourth Andalusian Health Plan; and Wales (United Kingdom) and the development of the Well-being of Future Generations Act 2015.

These case studies illustrate that a key requirement for socially sustainable development is to strengthen the social contract through a participatory planning and governance process. To achieve this, the principle of health in all policies must be applied, which means introducing health and well-being as the guiding principles in these governance processes. Broad participation in the core social arenas, the labour market, business, the educational system and the civic sector, by all groups and strata of the population will build social capital, which is the hallmark of a working social contract. It will lead to increased social inclusion, which in turn is a pre-requisite for decreasing the gap in social determinants of health and in its extension, reducing health inequities. This represents a major step towards a social investment paradigm, where health and well-being of the population is at the centre, both as an outcome of the investments and as the social and human capital, which could ensure future sustainable development in all its three main pillars: the economic, social and environmental.

I am very grateful for this opportunity to share these experiences, which I feel are an exemplary expression of WHO's strategy Health 2020. I hope it provides inspiration for those wishing to undertake similar measures at a regional level or beyond.

Ida Nilsson
Chair, Public Health Committee, Region Skåne, Sweden

Acknowledgments

The WHO Regional Office for Europe thanks members of Region Skåne, Sweden for their willingness to share their experiences with other countries and regions.

Special thanks go to the Urban Planning Department at Region Skåne, particularly to Richard Gullstrand (Assistant Head of Urban Planning Department), Therese Andersson (Head of Strategic Physical Planning Unit) and Sarah Ellström (Project Secretary) for the time they dedicated to being interviewed, their insight and the information they provided that helped make this publication possible.

Thanks go to Elisabeth Bengtsson (Head of Public Health Unit, Region Skåne), Monika Kosinska (Programme Manager, WHO Regional Office for Europe) and Per-Olof Östergren (Professor, Lund University, Sweden) for providing reviews of the publication in draft form and their guidance; Simone Tetz (Administrative Officer, WHO Regional Office for Europe) and Annalisa Buoro (Secretary, WHO Regional Office for Europe) for providing feedback on the first draft and on the overall structure of the publication; Margareta Rämgård (Senior Lecturer, Malmö University, Sweden) for providing information on participatory approaches; Mathias Grahn (Statistician, Region Skåne) and Sara Lindeberg (Specialist, Community Medicine, Region Skåne) for providing data from Region Skåne's public health surveys; and Kai Michelsen (Maastricht University, the Netherlands) and Mats Brandström (Public Health Strategist, Region Skåne) for their guidance.

The report was written by Clare Arvidsson (Project Assistant, Region Skåne), Francesco Zambon (Policy Officer, WHO Regional Office for Europe) and Per-Olof Östergren (Professor, Lund University, Sweden).

Special thanks go to the Region Skåne's Public Health and Social Sustainability Unit, Urban Planning Department, for providing the financial support for this publication.

The WHO Regional Office for Europe also thanks members of the Health Observatory, Department of Health and Social Solidarity, Autonomous Province of Trento, Italy; the Regional Ministry of Health of the Autonomous

Community of Andalusia, Spain; and Public Health Wales and the Welsh Government, United Kingdom; for contributing to the case studies in the publication. Particular thanks go to the following authors.

Autonomous Province of Trento, Italy

- Sara Carneri, Transparency and Participation Project, Trento, Italy
- Pirous Fateh-Moghadam, Health Observatory, Department of Health and Social Solidarity, Trento, Italy

Autonomous Community of Andalusia, Spain

- Ana Carriazo, General Secretariat of Public Health, Regional Ministry of Health, Government of Andalusia, Seville, Spain
- Alberto Fernández-Ajuria, Andalusian School of Public Health, Granada, Spain
- Manuel López, General Secretariat of Public Health, Regional Ministry of Health, Government of Andalusia, Seville, Spain
- Luis Andrés López-Fernández, Andalusian School of Public Health, Granada, Spain
- Josefa Ruiz, General Secretariat of Public Health, Regional Ministry of Health, Government of Andalusia, Seville, Spain

Wales, United Kingdom

- Sumina Azam, Consultant in Public Health, Policy, Research and International Development, Public Health Wales, Cardiff, United Kingdom
- Mark A. Bellis, Order of the British Empire, Director of Policy, Research and International Development, Public Health Wales, Cardiff, United Kingdom
- Mariana Dyakova, Consultant in Public Health, Policy, Research and International Development, Public Health Wales, Cardiff, United Kingdom
- Carolyn Lester, Principal Public Health Specialist, Policy, Research and International Development, Public Health Wales, Cardiff, United Kingdom
- Cathy Weatherup, Head of Health Inequalities and International Health, Welsh Government, Cardiff, United Kingdom

Executive summary

This publication documents the participatory process used by Region Skåne, Sweden to create the regional development strategy, *The open Skåne 2030*. It is based on the idea that the ultimate goal of all development is to improve the pre-requisites for the long-term survival and well-being of the population in a region, which entails action for increased social inclusion and a more equitable distribution of the social determinants of health. The publication also shares learning from the Autonomous Province of Trento's (Italy) development of a health plan; the Autonomous Community of Andalusia's (Spain) experience designing, implementing and assessing the Fourth Andalusian Health Plan; and the development of the Well-being of Future Generations Act 2015 in Wales (United Kingdom). It is produced in collaboration with the WHO Regions for Health Network, which supports the implementation of Health 2020, the WHO European policy for health and well-being.

The work with Skåne's regional development strategy has been, and will continue to be, a process that involves many actors, from state to local level and across all sectors. By actively working in this way, in multiple stages so as to include multiple actors and to gather input from ongoing initiatives, Skåne's regional development strategy has taken shape. This work has entailed creating a common foundation, as well as joint commitment to and shared responsibility for Skåne's development.

Skåne's regional development strategy has been focused on what needs to be done to strengthen Skåne's development in the mentioned perspective. *How* this is to be done is left to all development actors to reason out and develop. When all development actors in Skåne move in the same direction, Skåne's development potential can be fully utilized.

The following key messages could be useful to other regions, countries and municipalities that would like to adopt a similar participatory approach to tackle health inequalities and social sustainability.

Key messages

Find a common purpose for stakeholders and emphasize the potential of the common good.

Focus on the process rather than the product. Create ownership and involvement from all stakeholders.

Trust the process. Guide the process by being receptive and flowing with rather than controlling it.

Emphasize governance processes involving people and power over constructing a formal framework of structures.

Create ownership of the process through leadership and ambassadors.

Involve and empower other sectors (not only health).

Joint mobilization requires leadership characterized by courage and a willingness to take risks.

Do background analysis first in order to assess the characteristics of the situation.

Background

IMPLEMENTATION OF WHOLE-OF-GOVERNMENT AND WHOLE-OF-SOCIETY APPROACHES

While significant improvements in health and wealth have occurred in the WHO European Region, they have happened in an uneven and unequal fashion. In all European countries, good health and well-being is not equitably distributed across society. As evidenced by the *Review of social determinants and the health divide in the WHO European Region*, European countries face the challenge of remedying health effects arising from social gradients *(1)*. WHO's European health strategy, Health 2020 *(2)*, responds to this need. It allows for a re-thinking of priorities, a new focus on key determinants, strengthened leadership and a renewed approach to current governance mechanisms across all government sectors and society as a whole. Health 2020 has two strategic objectives that form the foundation of what it promotes.

First, **improve health for all and reduce health inequalities**. Health 2020 encourages governments to take actions to reduce health inequalities. This means acting on social determinants of health by means of interventions that address the most affected, address the social gradient in health directly, and are proportionate to the level of health and social need. It also calls for a rethinking of mechanisms, processes, relationships and institutional arrangements across all sectors. This includes encouraging public participation in policy-making and approaches that build up community resilience.

Second, **improve leadership and participatory governance for health**. Health 2020 also promotes collaborative leadership by means of innovative approaches to address behavioural determinants, the environment and health care issues. It recognizes the important role that advocacy and networking play in bringing many partners together, including empowerment of citizens by means of partnerships to know their rights and obtain what they need.

As health improvements cannot rely solely on the health sector, Health 2020 also calls for a whole-of-government and a whole-of-society approach that involves a range of stakeholders at all levels. It also has an equity focus suggesting new ways to identify important health gaps and focus individual and collective efforts on ways to reduce them.

This case study describes the participatory process taken by Region Skåne which, under Swedish legislation, has responsibility for regional development, and a permanent mandate from the Swedish state to coordinate regional development issues and to lead the work to draw up the regional development strategy. This strategy aims to formulate and create up to the year 2030 a broad joint approach to a common strategic objective that strengthens cooperation between different actors, and contributes to the creation of a context, a story, for those who live in Skåne, Sweden.

Skåne's regional development strategy, called *The open Skåne 2030 (3)*, is part of both national and European contexts, such as via the national strategy for regional growth and attractiveness *(3)*, the European Union (EU) Strategy for the Baltic Sea Region *(4)*, WHO's Health 2020 strategy *(2)*, Europe 2020 *(5)*, the EU's energy and climate goals for 2030 *(6)* and the EU's cohesion policy *(7)*.

Skåne's regional development strategy is also integrated with many other processes and strategies that together provide a direction for the future development work at both regional and local levels. Examples include *An international innovation strategy for Skåne 2012–2020 (8)*, *Strategies for the polycentric Skåne (9)*, the transport services programme, regional mobilization around new research facilities, Region Skåne's business development platform for recruitment needs and training, the equal opportunities strategy for Skåne, public health campaigns, the strategic environmental programme, the climate and energy strategy for Skåne, the rural programme, transport infrastructure planning, nongovernmental organization (NGO) sector collaboration, the culture plan and municipal comprehensive land-use plans *(3)*.

In line with Health 2020, the local council of Region Skåne committed itself to establishing a process, with an aim to achieve more sustainable growth and greater appeal for Skåne, which involved a wide range of stakeholders and supported intersectoral problem solving. The process encouraged effective leadership throughout society, and empowered stakeholders and citizens.

An important factor was Region Skåne's commitment to standing back and trusting that the participatory process would produce the best-informed joint decisions for Skåne's future and, from a public health point of view, that the health and well-being of Skåne's citizens would be prioritized. With their combined size working towards an open Skåne by 2030, these joint stakeholders are able to exert a great deal of influence and create enormous possibilities for transformation.

This publication makes a key contribution to the Regions for Health Network. With the Göteborg Manifesto (10), endorsed in 2012, the Network positions itself as an effective and unique cooperation platform for Health 2020 implementation at the subnational level. The Network fosters exchanges of experience, best practice and lessons learnt centred around the design of policies focusing on environmental, social and economic determinants and tackling health inequities.

Regions are usually very active and proactive players. They are quick, dynamic learners too. It is generally acknowledged that the most durable lessons learnt come from example. Publications like this one are, in this sense, useful points of reference. They teach through example and provide inspiration, which may motivate other regions to take similar actions.

A THEORETICAL FRAMEWORK

Developing societies demand bottom-up processes. No actor can own, lead or steer a system. Instead, there is the need to co-create, by focusing on issue-driven development, where each actor's capabilities are used to solve a common problem, rather than sector-driven development. Legislation in Sweden (Law 2010:630 on regional development responsibility in certain counties) states that the responsible regional development actor should involve municipalities and state-level actors in the process of creating the regional development strategy. For a number of years, multilevel governance has been in focus, where the interactions between different geographic spheres have been the main issue. Region Skåne's regional development strategy used a whole-of-government approach, where the interaction between different stakeholders is needed to create change. In this way, Region Skåne decided to adopt a participatory approach for the creation of its joint strategic plan.

The emergence of (the concept of) new public health is the position that the ultimate goal of human society must be to guarantee the long-term survival and well-being of the human species, in other words a sustainable future development *(11)*. The report of the Brundtland Commission, *Report of the World Commission on Environment and Development: our common future*, defined three pillars of sustainable development: economic, social and environmental *(12)*. These pillars are inseparably interlinked. Building a society that secures social sustainability, therefore, has crucial implications for the other two pillars of sustainability. The issue of social sustainability is of crucial concern for overall sustainability.

Since long-term survival and well-being almost perfectly matches the WHO definition of health *(13)*, challenges to social sustainability are also challenges to the health of a certain population. One such major challenge is the issue of social exclusion, which underlies the issue of social equity. That is to say, the mechanisms that drive social exclusion are also the drivers of social inequity and, accordingly, are expressed as health inequities in a given society. An obvious strategy to counter social exclusion in a society is to increase the participatory mechanisms in the governance of the development processes of that society. This requires a focus on the groups and individuals who are most at risk for social exclusion, so this becomes an empowerment process. However, in order not to be a token project, this should apply to the main development processes in a society, and all relevant stakeholders should take part. This can guarantee a positive development in social capital and strengthens the social contract, which is the foundation of societal function. Thus, issues of societal development and health are intimately linked together, as can be implicitly understood by the concept of health in all policies, the cornerstone of WHO's new overarching policy Health 2020 advocating for a better and more equitable health development in Europe *(2)*.

Participatory approaches to health research are increasingly drawing attention. The International Collaboration for Participatory Health Research (ICPHR) explains that, while the approaches come from broad social movements striving for a more democratic and inclusive society, great diversity exists among them in terms of intention, theory, process and outcome.

The ICPHR position paper *(14)* explains that, in the absence of a definitive description of the participatory health research (PHR) approach, an international discussion exists:

> *The goal of PHR is to maximize the participation of those whose life or work is the subject of the research in all stages of the research process. Such participation is the core, defining principle of PHR, setting this type of research apart from other approaches in the health field. Research is not done 'on' people as passive subjects providing 'data' but 'with' them to provide relevant information for improving their lives. The entire research process is viewed as a partnership between stakeholders which may include academic researchers; professionals in the fields of health care, education and social welfare; members of civil society; policy-makers and others (14).*

Table 1 summarizes the common distinguishing features of participatory approaches to health research. Clearly, the intentional consequences go far beyond the health sector and more into the realm of creating positive sustainable social change. Through the engagement of stakeholders, recognizing the value of each person's contribution to the process is not only practical, but also collaborative and empowering in finding solutions together. Of course, many different perspectives are given and assumptions are challenged; but this enables the creation of a space for new transformative insights offering fresh approaches.

The ability of a broad coalition of stakeholders to address the social and political factors that impinge on the group as a whole also widens the impact of the process. Through the communication of the essence of the intervention, others can deem if it is relevant to their situation.

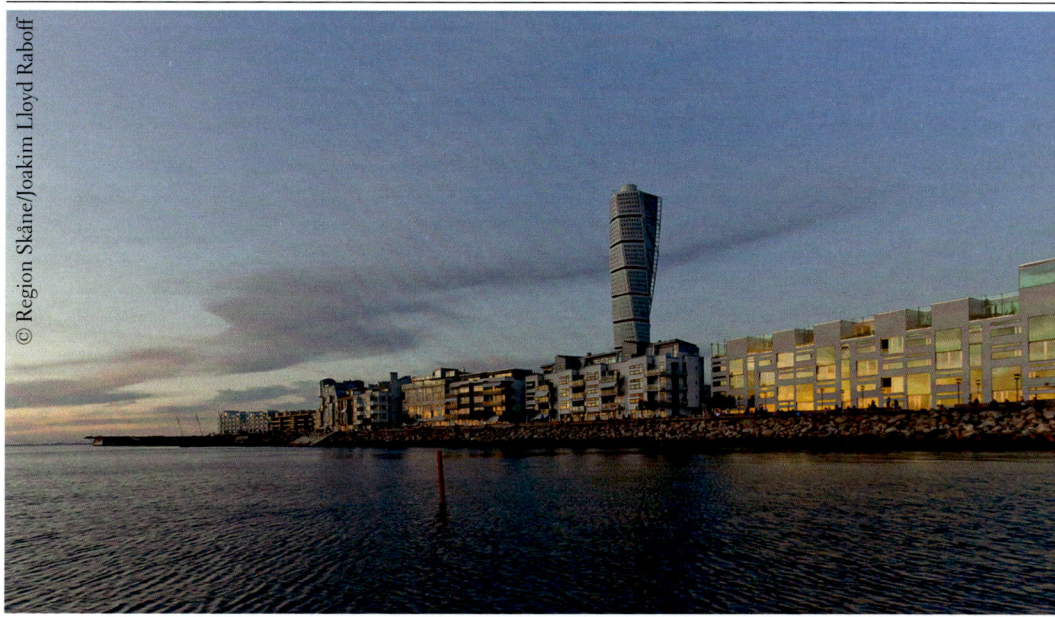

© Region Skåne/Joakim Lloyd Raboff

Background

Table 1. Summary of common distinguishing features of participatory approaches to health research

Characteristics of PHR	Description
Participatory	• Maximize the active participation of those whose life or work is the subject of the research in all stages of the research process. • Provide the opportunity for all participants to be equitably involved to the maximum degree possible throughout the research. • Maximizing participation requires an active and intensive commitment on the part of those initiating the research. • The process is viewed as a partnership between stakeholders. • The co-creative process requires facilitation, and the building and maintenance of trust.
Locally situated	• The issue being researched must be located in the social system, which is likely to adopt the changes that result from the research process. • Emphasize local level of knowledge and experience without requiring a local scope; statements can be made about issues at regional, national or international level.
Collective research process	• The process is conducted by a group representing the various stakeholders including engaged citizens, NGOs, health professionals, academic researchers and policy-makers.
Collectively owned	• Ownership of the research lies in the hands of the group conducting the study.
Aims for transformation and social change	• Aim to create positive social change as a result of the research process for those whose life or work is the focus of the research. • Enable participants to recognize their current situation and how to be involved in finding solutions. • Promote empowerment through enabling people to take an active, deciding role in all aspects of the research process. • Contribute to sustainable change beyond the span of the research project, for example, by involving a broad coalition of stakeholders and setting up structures for sustained learning and action.

Characteristics of PHR	Description
Promotes critical reflexivity	• Consider how power and powerlessness affect the daily lives and practice of those whose life or work is the focus of the research. • Require professionals to question their roles and knowledge based on power differentials between them and service users. • Act together with others to address the social and political factors that impinge on the group as a whole.
Produces knowledge that is local, collective, co-created, dialogical and diverse	• Provide the opportunity for people to articulate their local knowledge about the subject at hand based on their direct experience. • Knowledge is produced in an ongoing dialogue among participants on all aspects of the research process. • Uncover and examine different points of view and potentially present differences in perspectives. • Recognize that knowledge is always in a process of becoming and is never fixed. • This approach requires facilitation so that trust can be built and maintained.
Strives for a broad impact	• Aim to bring about social change. • This process includes a continual cycle of look, reflect and act. • Recognizing and articulating impact over time is difficult.
Produces local evidence based on a broad understanding of generalizability	• Develop interventions for a specific time and place, and give primacy to the local context in order to produce local evidence. • Obtain a deep understanding of the essence of a situation that can be communicated to others who can then judge the relevance of the findings for their own situation *(15)*.
Follows specific validity criteria	• Incorporate both qualitative and quantitative research methods. • Importance is placed on the adherence to validity criteria such as participatory, intersubjective and ethical validity.

Table 1 contd

Characteristics of PHR	Description
Dialectical process characterized by messiness	• This is characterized by dialogues of different perspectives often resulting in several different views on the issue at hand. • The dialogical process intends to promote transformational learning making possible new, transformative insights offering fresh approaches. • The process defies a simple linear description of planning and implementing a research project. Rather, a spiral pattern unfolds, where participants reflect, plan, act and observe in several repeating cycles (16). • Conflict is created for many participants as their assumptions are questioned. A so-called messiness arises in the process creating a communicative space to deconstruct current beliefs and construct new ideas.

Source: What is participatory health research? *(14)*.

Setting the scene

KEY FACTS ABOUT SKÅNE

Skåne is a county in the southernmost region of Sweden and part of the transnational Öresund region,[1] connecting to Copenhagen, Denmark by a road and rail bridge and by ferries. The biggest city in Skåne is Malmö.

Skåne has a population of 1.27 million (13% of Sweden's total) *(17)* and a total area of just over 11 000 km^2 (3% of Sweden's total area) *(18)*. Nearly one fifth of its population is born overseas, coming from 193 countries *(3)*.

Skåne is divided into 33 municipalities with 13 cities, three national parks and over 200 nature reserves *(18)*. The landscape is varied with close proximity to the sea, beaches, forests, farmland and plains.

REGION SKÅNE

Region Skåne is responsible for:

- health care and medical services including primary, specialist, ambulance and dental care;
- public transportation including a cross-regional and cross-national train system (Öresundståg); and
- regional growth and development – national and EU development, urban planning, and infrastructure and environmental and cultural matters – and, together with the municipalities, tourism.

Region Skåne receives funds from regional taxes (65%), government subsidies (19%), patient contributions (3%) and other sources (13%).

Skåne has been growing for many years. This positive trend brings many opportunities and also many challenges. This selection of facts

---

[1] Öresund region consists of southern Sweden and eastern Denmark.

about Skåne are based on the Organisation for Economic Co-operation and Development's (OECD's) review of Skåne *(19)*, together with comprehensive material and published reports and statistics, and presented in *The open Skåne 2030 (3)*.

- Skåne has a young, varied and growing population.
- Many of Skåne's residents are living longer.
- Skåne's inhabitants are becoming healthier but differences in social determinants of health are increasing.
- Sweden is tolerant, but intolerance is greater in Skåne than in the rest of the country.

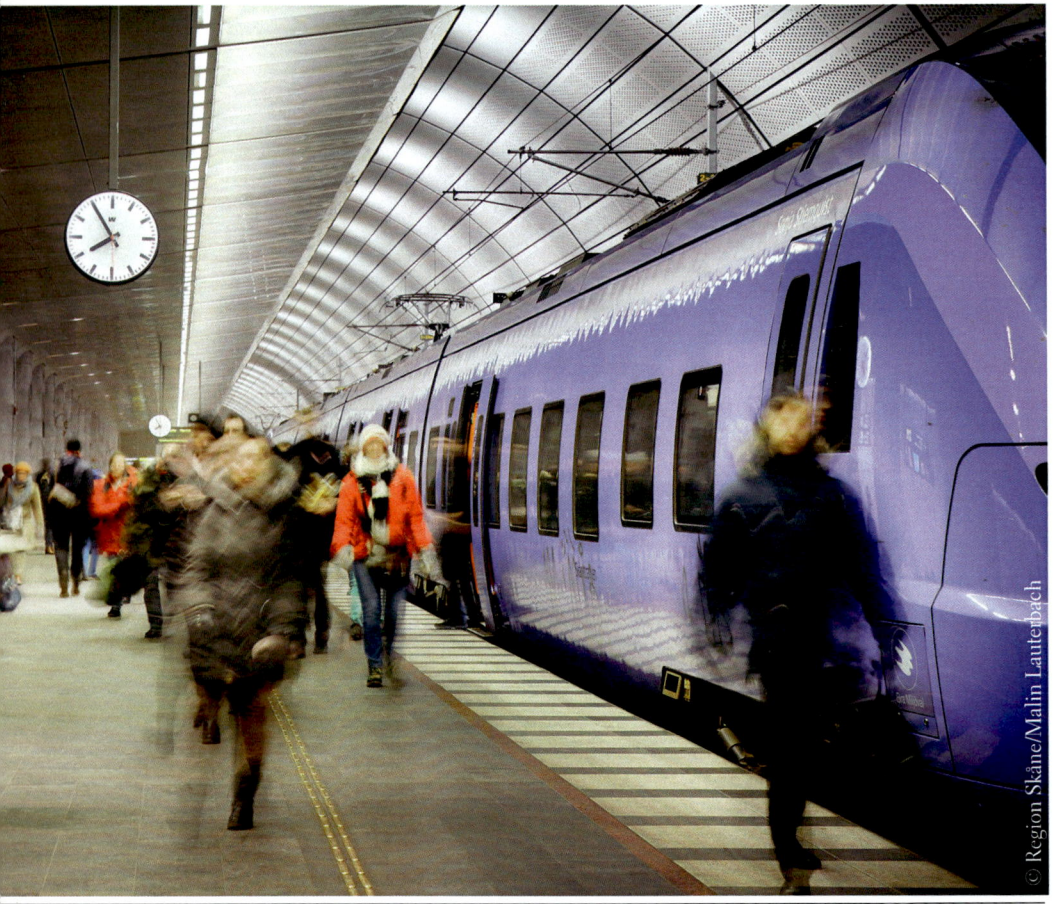

- The level of education is high, while too few qualify for secondary school.
- Too few are in work, even if demand for employees is great.
- Skåne has two labour market regions with poor mobility within and between them.
- Skåne exhibits strong innovation but needs more viable and growing companies.
- Skåne has low productivity and taxable capacity.
- Skåne has low growth.
- Skåne has a polycentric urban structure that is unique in Sweden.
- Skåne is the link to the continent, but integration in the Öresund region has lost momentum.
- Skåne is a transit region and more investments in communications are needed.
- Skåne has beautiful natural surroundings and Europe's best farmland.
- Skåne faces major environmental challenges (3).

Skåne's agenda

> Region Skåne has, under Swedish legislation on regional development responsibility, a permanent mandate from the Swedish state to coordinate regional development issues and to head the work to draw up the regional development strategy. A decisive success factor is that this work is conducted openly, inclusively and with continual dialogue. Skåne's inhabitants, municipalities, authorities, colleges and universities, trade and industry, and the idea-based sector need to participate if more initiatives, collaborations and networks are to arise, and if Skåne is to achieve more sustainable growth and greater appeal (3).

In addition to the national mandate supporting the opportunity for a joint regional strategy, Region Skåne's understanding of the role of a region was changing. There was an awareness of the new geographical models for nations, regions and municipalities; the increasing internationalization where regions were expected to act globally; and the importance of taking a cross-border perspective, for example, to Skåne's neighbours Copenhagen,

Denmark and Hamburg, Germany. This set the scene for the discussions that took place within the region and are clearly seen in the priority areas in the regional development strategy.

In terms of the economic climate for the regional strategy work, Region Skåne felt that using its own budget was important. However, it recognized the economic potential in applying for funding from the EU structural funds for further projects that could be carried out in the municipalities.

In the autumn of 2010, following an OECD territorial review of Sweden (20), Region Skåne decided to carry out a similar review specifically of Skåne (19), which initiated the work with its regional development strategy (3). The *OECD territorial reviews: Skåne, Sweden 2012* evaluated the challenges and opportunities faced by Skåne, and highlighted where Skåne should focus in the coming years (19). It addressed questions such as where is the potential and competitiveness? Are there resources which could be used better? How should all of Skåne's actors work together to reach common goals? How can innovation be strengthened in the whole of Skåne? How can prosperity increase?

The OECD review of Skåne, which took two years to complete, based its analysis on three of Europe 2020's flagship initiatives – innovation, environment and the labour market (5). During the process, OECD carried out many consultations with the municipality, the County Administrative Board of Skåne, the business sector, NGOs and the Swedish Association of Local Authorities and Regions. This provided a useful starting point for Region Skåne's discussions with its stakeholders for the regional strategy work. While not explicitly recommending the use of a participatory approach, OECD stresses the need to engage many actors and cross-cutting approaches.

The analysis and recommendations reached by OECD provided both a clear and concrete proposal for how Region Skåne could make the most of Skåne's full potential and achieve its vision of improving the quality of life for all its citizens (Box 1). It also became an extremely effective tool for discussion in the strategy process.

Box 1. Summary of OECD's assessments and recommendations for Skåne

- The way forward is about the opportunity of a growing population, strong innovation architecture and a healthy environment to enhance growth.
- Skåne should be promoted as a smart and healthy place to live, work and visit.
- A successful region, Skåne must nevertheless overcome a number of challenges to realize its potential.
- Population inflows mean that Skåne must run to stand still, that is, "has had to generate stronger aggregate growth than most regions just to keep per capita GDP [gross domestic product] rising" *(19)*.
- Skåne can do more to use its innovation strengths to enhance growth and employment generation.
- Better monitoring and evaluation are needed to support evidence-based implementation.
- Skåne can do more to promote trans-cluster and cross-border innovation.
- Greater private sector involvement in the innovation system is needed.
- Skåne should pursue a dual-track innovation strategy.
- Labour-market policies must be seen as a key component of structural growth policy.
- More can be done to realize migrants' potential contribution to Skåne's prosperity.
- More can be done to facilitate school-to-work transitions among youth.
- Skåne could benefit from expanded labour markets.

Source: OECD territorial reviews: Skåne, Sweden 2012 (19).

Open Skåne 2030: the process

INTERNAL PROCESS

Creativity

Region Skåne has a history of regional development strategies, 1999–2004, 2004–2009, 2009–2016 *(21)* and the current strategy 2014–2030 *(3)*:

> With Skåne's current strategy, disruptive models were needed to understand the irrational processes that occur in society. An aspect of the participatory approach is that it defies a simple linear description of planning and implementing a research project. Rather, a spiral pattern unfolds, where participants reflect, plan, act and observe in several repeating cycles *(16)*. Region Skåne saw the new strategy as something about creating interaction and movement. The focus was on the actors and processes moving around in a continuous mutual interaction; these movements create new conditions and opportunities, new ideas and collaborations – and hence new movement – the eco-system in motion.

More simply, Region Skåne knew it did not want another so-called product for its regional strategy, especially as many processes and projects were already running without any elaborate strategies. Region Skåne wanted to focus on the process or processes rather than the product, and keep it alive and dynamic, as well as connected to the OECD report on Skåne *(19)*. One premise of the participatory approach is about producing knowledge that is ongoing and never fixed; "knowledge is always in a process of becoming" *(14)*.

To be able to work across sectors and through systems, Region Skåne wanted to guide the process by flowing with it and being receptive rather than controlling it. It saw its role as a sounding board – a player that moved in-between stakeholders like a free agent, a broker or convener.

Through the years, Region Skåne has considered using a logical framework approach, which is an instrument for logical analysis and structured thinking in project planning *(22)*. The Swedish Agency for International Development Cooperation (Sida) and other donor agencies encourage its use as an instrument to improve the planning, implementation, monitoring and evaluation of a development intervention. Sida writes that the systematic application of the method, with good judgement and sound common sense, can help to improve the quality, and hence the relevance, feasibility and sustainability of development cooperation *(22)*.

In the previous regional strategy (2009–2016) *(21)*, objectives and activities were set out in sector programmes such as infrastructure; traffic; and workplace, environmental and public health promotion programmes. In other words, sectors were working in silos rather than being synchronized. Region Skåne wanted to challenge this multilevel governance model and achieve a whole-of-government approach that was more systematic and cohesive with the new regional development strategy.

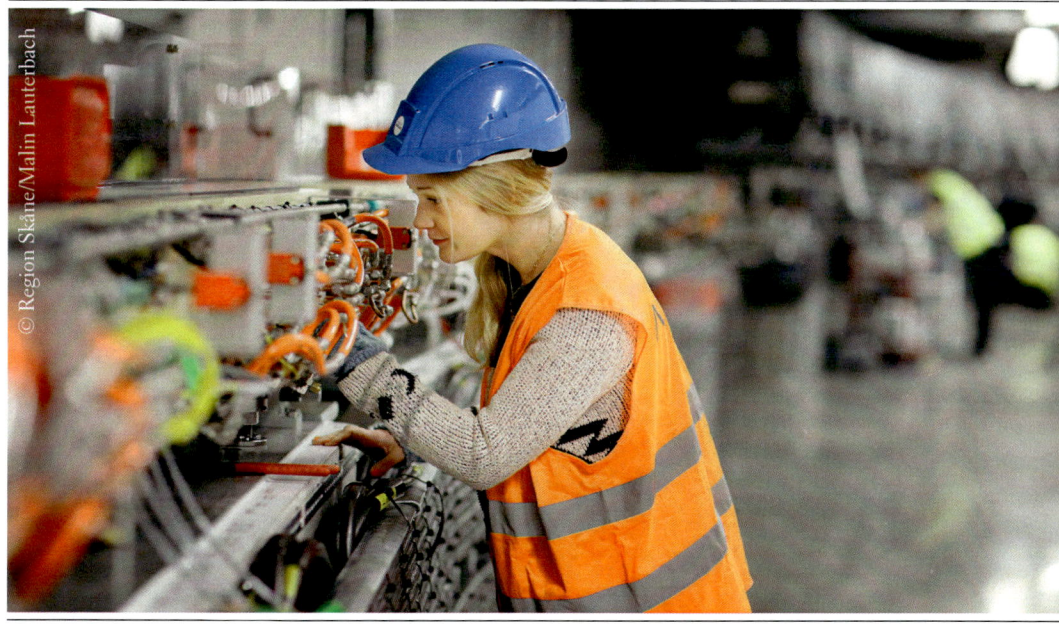

Input

Region Skåne's strategy project group wanted to use the many existing strategies (including six listed below) that had been regionally agreed as a starting point for its regional development work. It also wanted to harness this energy coming from Skåne and connect it to the internal process.

The commissioning of an **OECD territorial review of Skåne** *(19)* initiated the work of Skåne's regional development strategy. Using an independent and

Open Skåne 2030: the process

influential body gave more credibility and importance to the review findings. The review required many consultations and kick-started the process of gathering stakeholders. The review's analysis and recommendations provided a clear and concrete proposal for how Region Skåne could make the most of Skåne's full potential, and achieve its vision of improving the quality of life for all its citizens.

Regional analyses from ongoing processes and collaborative projects between Region Skåne and Skåne's municipalities, and follow-up from previous regional development strategies were also used as input.

In Skåne, two large research facilities, the European Spallation Source (ESS) and MAX IV will be ready in 2015 and 2019 respectively. The purpose of **TITA** – the acronym for the Swedish words for **growth, innovation, accessibility and attractiveness** – is to stimulate growth and strengthen the innovation, accessibility and attractiveness of the south Swedish county of Skåne, based on the establishment of these facilities. The project consisted of several parts focusing on different aspects of the impact that the research installations will and can have on regional development in southern Sweden. One example is relocation support for the establishment of companies and their employees in the county (23).

For physical planning to be sustainable for the whole of Skåne, a regional perspective and collaboration between all parties are required. In 2005, to successfully manage future growth, the municipalities of Skåne and Region Skåne developed a joint knowledge-bank within the **Structural picture of Skåne** (24). This is an ongoing arena for dialogue around regional development regarding physical planning and takes into account, for example, the development of attractive living environments and places where people will want to live and work.

Within Region Skåne there is a continual and ongoing dialogue around how **Region Skåne** and Skåne as a **brand** are marketed in national and international contexts. The project group for the regional development work took these discussions into consideration.

The Swedish Government requested Region Skåne to identify **seven top-priority challenges** in Skåne. This process contributed to the regional development work.

Ownership

The previous regional strategy *(21)* involved only a small number of people at Region Skåne who steered the process. This time, Region Skåne wanted to involve representatives at different levels in different sectors to really create internal ownership of the project. In the spring of 2012, Region Skåne secured the role of process manager and agreed on three levels of involvement internally.

- The **Political Steering Group** consisted of nine top-level politicians from Region Skåne. Region Skåne felt that politicians would be best placed for this role in order to create ownership and ambassadorship, and wanted people who would develop a personal connection to the process and drive it forward.

- The **Regional Development Steering Group** was a non-political group that included the Regional Development Director at Region Skåne. Ideally, it could have had even wider representation and attempted to have more presence at the Board of Directors.

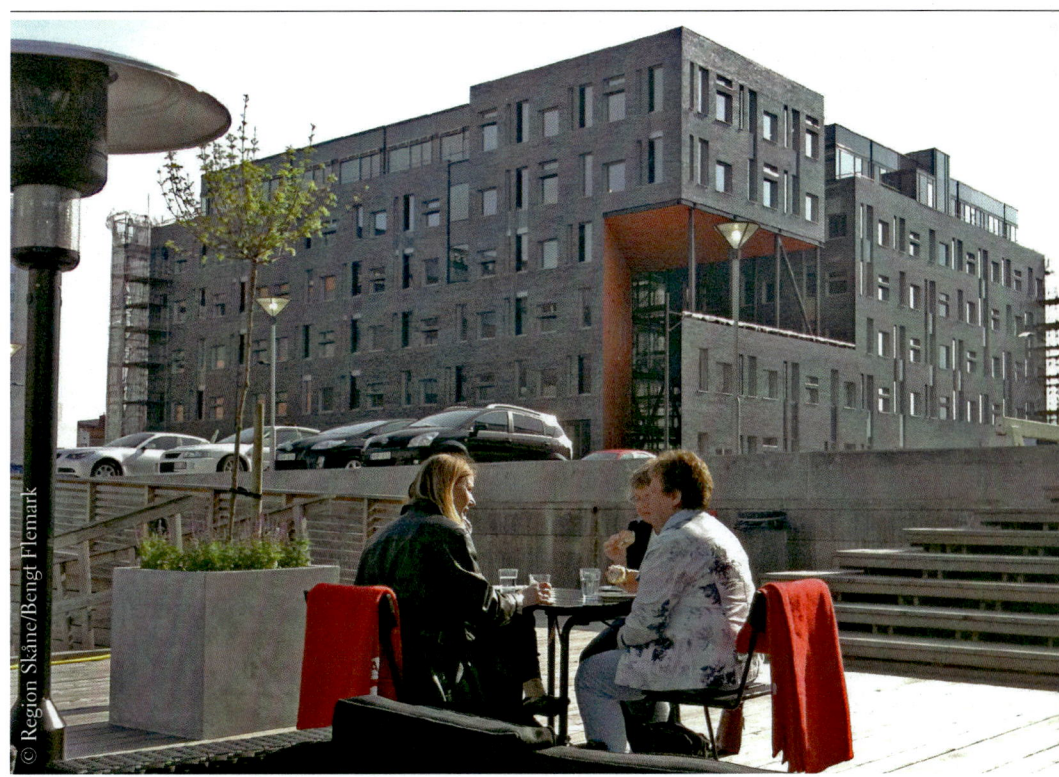

Open Skåne 2030: the process

- The **Process Group** worked at the functional level and included the process manager and 7–10 people from all parts of Region Skåne.

In addition, an OECD advisory group, external consultants who facilitated many of the dialogues, and a communication consultancy firm who designed the layout of the product and the website also participated.

One outcome from the many discussions between Region Skåne and the politicians was that the regional development strategy would be predominantly for municipalities and businesses, rather than for Skåne's citizens. This can be seen in its language and approach, although its focus is ultimately on the citizen's welfare and quality of life. Fig. 1 depicts the timeline used in the process.

Fig. 1. Timeline used in the process

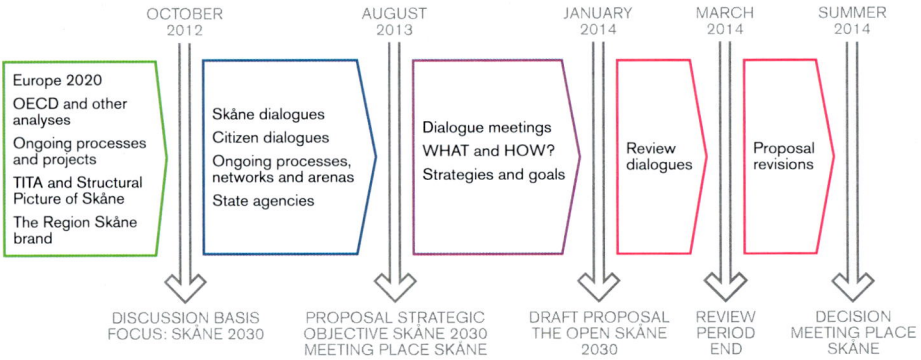

Source: adapted and reproduced with permission from Region Skåne *(3).*

External process

Skåne Dialogues

During the autumn of 2012 and spring 2013, Region Skåne implemented the Skåne Dialogues – dialogues with Skåne's 33 municipalities about the vision for an open Skåne 2030. This fundamental part of the process took one and a half years to complete. Leading politicians with representatives of Region Skåne's strategy project group visited each of the 33 municipal executive boards to identify important issues concerning Skåne's future and to discuss the work of a regional development strategy. The ambition was to create a joint picture of the current situation, and to determine which challenges and opportunities Skåne faced.

Prior to the Skåne Dialogues, Region Skåne sent out preparatory material that combined important issues with facts about Skåne. It contained a scenario analysis where four different extreme and exaggerated scenarios were imagined for the future of Skåne. The purpose was to stimulate discussion about the future of Skåne and the challenges that would be met on the way.

Region Skåne used the same material when it held parallel discussions with other collaborative partners such as state agencies, universities and colleges, business and trade organizations, idea-based organizations, projects and networks.

The findings from the municipal and dialogue meetings gave rise to a proposal document that creates a picture, a tale, for those who live in Skåne 2030. It is divided into six themes: Skåne has a pulse; is for everyone; is global; has jobs; is healthy; and is in balance.

These ideas are in the final version of *The open Skåne 2030 (3)*. In the summer of 2013, Region Skåne presented the proposal at a conference event Meeting Place Skåne.

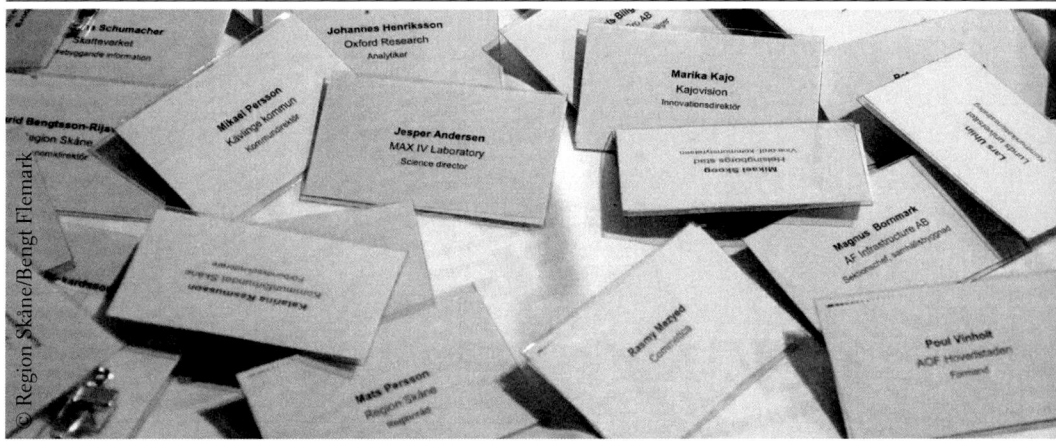

Refinement

The stakeholders that Region Skåne invited to the Meeting Place Skåne were the development actors in Skåne who would be responsible for carrying out the regional development work (Box 2). This same group was involved throughout the whole process.

> **Box 2. Meeting Place Skåne**
>
> The **aim** was to strengthen involvement and participation with Skåne's regional development strategy *The open Skåne 2030* and gather actors from different sectors to discuss Skåne's important future issues together.
>
> The **target group** comprised:
>
> - civil servants and politicians from Region Skåne and all of Skåne's 33 municipalities;
> - all public authorities;
> - a mix of private and public organizations;
> - all colleges and universities;
> - the business sector – those who participated in Region Skåne business networks;
> - NGOs who participated in Region Skåne networks;
> - all unions; and
> - actors from Öresund (Copenhagen, Denmark and Skåne region) and the neighbouring regions in Sweden.
>
> The **timeline** covered two years.
>
> - In August 2013, a proposal document on open Skåne was presented.
> - In August 2014, *The open Skåne 2030* was presented.
> - In August 2015, more in-depth work took place with the regional development strategy and collaborations were strengthened.
>
> Some **key facts** summarize the event.
>
> - Region Skåne was the host of the one-day event.
> - Thirty-five seminars took place in which half were arranged by actors outside Region Skåne including the municipalities, authorities, businesses and NGOs.
> - It provided an opportunity to mingle, debate politics and celebrate.
> - In 2014, 1300 people attended and a similar number were expected to attend in 2015.
> - All activities took place at Region Skåne's offices in Malmö in close proximity to stimulate conversation, spontaneity and flexibility.

During the autumn of 2013, Region Skåne held six one-day conferences, one for each theme from the proposal document. It invited the same target group as the Meeting Place Skåne, nearly 3000 people from Skåne's 33 municipalities, public authorities and organizations, the business sector, colleges and universities, NGOs, unions and individuals. On average, 60 participants attended each meeting whose purpose was to refine the proposal, and identify possible strategies and interventions. This time, facilitators led the process, which helped build and maintain trust among the stakeholders.

Fig.2 shows how the consultation process was dynamic and constantly changing. Region Skåne was the actor that guided the process and the voices towards an end goal.

Fig. 2. A dynamic process

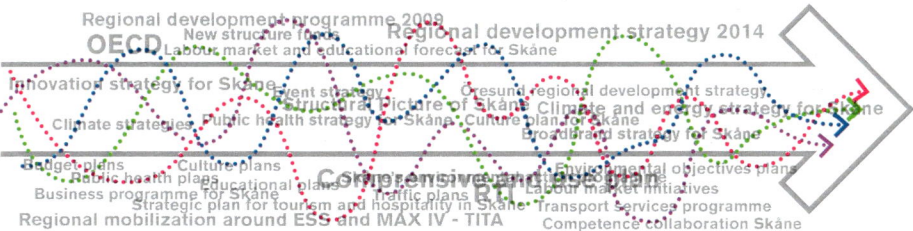

Source: adapted and reproduced with permission from Region Skåne (3).

REVIEW PERIOD

Region Skåne circulated the draft proposal for a new regional development strategy for review from January to March 2014. It encouraged approximately 120 formal stakeholders and 3500 people affiliated with Skåne's development work to submit comments on the draft. A website also enabled other interested parties to submit their opinions *(25)*.

Over 100 official organizations and a few private individuals submitted formal replies on the draft proposal. Region Skåne published all submitted opinions on its website for all to access.

During the review period, Region Skåne involved Skåne's citizens in a public dialogue (the citizen dialogues) with facilitators carrying out discussions.

- Focus group discussions took place on the five prioritized standpoints in the draft proposal. Although they were open to all, mostly older people took part and no further effort was made to include unrepresented groups.
- Discussions in secondary school scenarios focused on tolerance aspects within the draft proposal.

Further citizen involvement involved the Skåne panel, an existing e-panel representative of Skåne's citizens comprising almost 4000 people. Region Skåne implements regular citizen surveys through the Skåne panel as part of its work with public dialogue. With this study, it wanted to investigate citizen's attitudes about the objectives within the five prioritized areas they considered the most important to the development of Skåne.

The study was carried out via the internet (three respondents were contacted by telephone as they could not respond via the internet), and a reminder was sent out. The response rate was 74% and showed significant differences between groups based on sex, age, employment, education level and region. Around one third of responders gave highest priority to the standpoint that the health of the Skåne's population in 2030 would have improved and the differences would have decreased as regards equality. Almost equal priority was given to the standpoint that more Skåne citizens would be satisfied with their lives.

Region Skåne continued to work with its target audience, including municipalities, public agencies, trade organizations, industry and NGOs, in the review period by conducting a number of dialogues to discuss the proposal. It also visited individual municipalities for more in-depth discussions and arranged meetings with other actors who requested them.

Summaries from different review dialogues and submitted opinions provided the basis for revisions made to the development strategy. This resulted in a strengthened proposal in the areas where most comments were received.

In order to provide feedback on the opinions submitted during the review period and discuss how to make Skåne more attractive, Region Skåne invited those interested to a one-day conference, Skåne's Appeal, in April 2014. The conference also highlighted how the strategy work linked to the national strategy for regional growth and attractiveness. Around 200 people from the target group attended (Box 2).

Adoption

In June 2014, the Region Skåne Executive Committee decided unanimously to adopt the regional development strategy, *The open Skåne 2030 (3)*, which was the result of extensive dialogue with citizens, civil society, business and the public sector.

The aim is to achieve an open Skåne by 2030 through five prioritized standpoints that start from the individual and extend outwards towards the system and aim to strengthen Skåne in a number of areas. Skåne shall:

- offer optimism and quality of life
- be a strong, sustainable growth engine
- benefit from its polycentric urban structure
- develop the welfare services of tomorrow
- be globally attractive.

Implementation – moving from what to how

> *The decisions made today will shape the Skåne of tomorrow. Skåne's regional development strategy aims to provide direction for the ongoing development work in Skåne. Taking a stand on where Skåne is to be in the future makes it easier to make the right decisions and find the right forms of collaboration. However, words, willingness and ambition must be backed up by actions. And all development actors in Skåne must contribute (3).*

For the open Skåne to become a reality, everyone must contribute. Skåne's regional development strategy has been focused on *what* needs to be done to strengthen Skåne's development. *How* this is to be done is left to all development actors to reason out and develop. Strategies and action plans that work intersectorally and collaboratively among the development actors are needed. Combining social processes with economic growth is also needed, for example, addressing the issues of environmental sustainability in relation to industrial processes. When all development actors in Skåne move in the same direction, Skåne's development potential can be fully utilized.

Continued dialogue is central to implementation to enable the necessary joint involvement and joint actions to happen. This will entail different actors

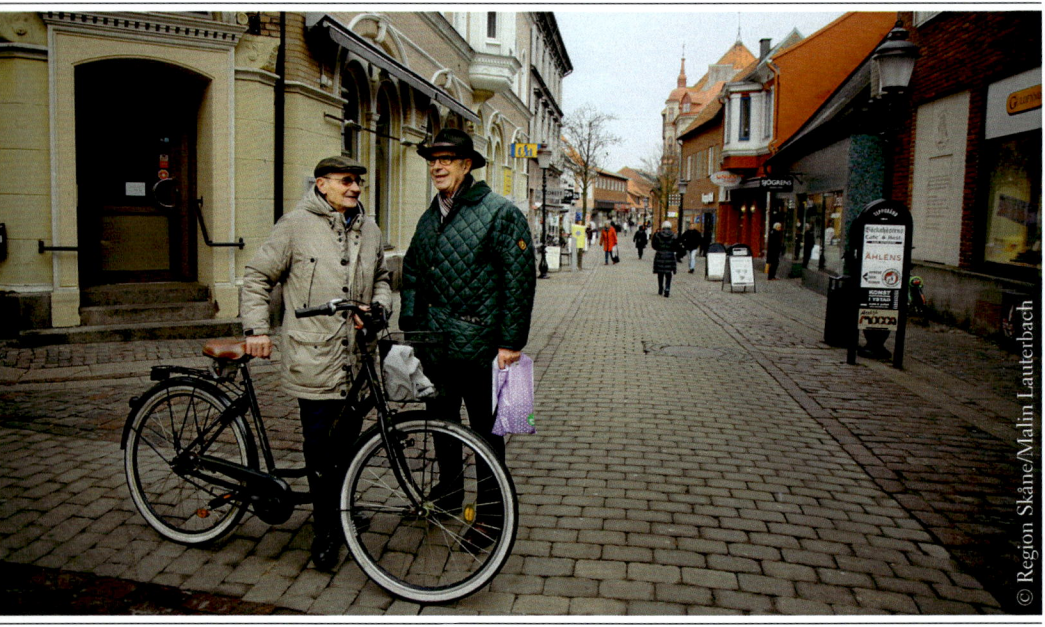

taking the helm in their areas of responsibility and working actively with new initiatives.

Work with Skåne's development will also require skills development, refined leadership and ambassadorships so that all development actors assimilate the strategic objective. Human and social capital are essential, and hence necessary to provide skills on how to be and achieve a mind-set of a free agent (or broker or convener). In the autumn of 2015, Region Skåne plans to offer an internal programme (under development) for 15–20 leaders on how to navigate in a world of change.

Furthermore, Region Skåne will assume responsibility for the implementation of the development strategy within its areas of responsibility, such as budgets, operational plans and communication work. For example, in line with the EU agenda Europe 2020 (5), Region Skåne is open to using external financial instruments, such as the EU structural funds, in order to finance parts of the implementation.

Region Skåne will offer special arenas for all actors involved in the development strategy to meet, such as Meeting Place Skåne and Skåne's Appeal. Moreover, a website will act as a digital platform for everyone working to realize the strategic objective (25).

PUBLIC HEALTH

WHO's European health strategy, Health 2020 (2), provides the overarching goal for the Public Health and Social Sustainability Unit at Region Skåne. The objectives of Health 2020 are to significantly improve population health and well-being, reduce health inequalities and ensure people-centred systems that are universal, equal and of high quality. WHO recommends taking a cross-sectoral and preventive approach, and addressing the root causes of health problems from a life-course perspective. To achieve these goals, new leadership tools based on the social determinants of health, equity and sustainability are needed (2).

Health 2020 emphasizes the many determinants of health and that the traditional health sector cannot be solely responsible to work towards equality in health. The aim is to achieve health in all policies whereby all decision-makers are responsible to think about the health effects in relation to their respective policy areas. Cooperative efforts based on shared objectives and common priorities are essential (2).

Region Skåne's *The open Skåne 2030* (3) replaces previous regional public health strategies developed in collaboration with municipalities, as the public health perspective is now integrated throughout the regional development strategy. Health and well-being are particularly emphasized as the first of five prioritized standpoints: Skåne shall offer optimism and quality of life:

> *Skåne's population is thriving and living increasingly longer, but many people's lives are limited by ill health, unemployment and alienation. The aim is for all people to enjoy the basic conditions necessary to shape their lives and to participate in and contribute to society to the best of their ability (3).*

This standpoint has several substrategies.

- Strengthen individual spirit and freedom.
- Create the conditions for all people to have the means to shape their own life.
- Enhance the opportunities for lifelong learning.
- Strengthen entrepreneurship and individual innovation.
- Use culture to support development.
- Work for improved and more equal health.
- Create sustainable and attractive living environments.
- Ensure that Skåne thrives.

From the vision of *The open Skåne 2030* (3), the Public Health and Social Sustainability Unit produced a joint action plan (26) whose purpose is to develop the social sustainability perspective, and focus on increased equities in health as an important measure for social sustainability. Occupation, education, accommodation, trust, social networks, culture, the environment and climate are all examples of important social sustainability factors for health in the population.

The action plan focuses on creating better coordinated public health work within and between units in Region Skåne, and aims to create better conditions for collaboration between activities. The public health department also firmly establishes that Region Skåne, who is not solely responsible for the whole of public health work in Skåne, is but one of many actors in Skåne together with municipalities, public authorities, the business sector, NGOs and universities. With the action plan as a base for organizational-wide work, Region Skåne aims to stimulate and develop collaboration with other actors that want to work for better and more equal health in the population of Skåne.

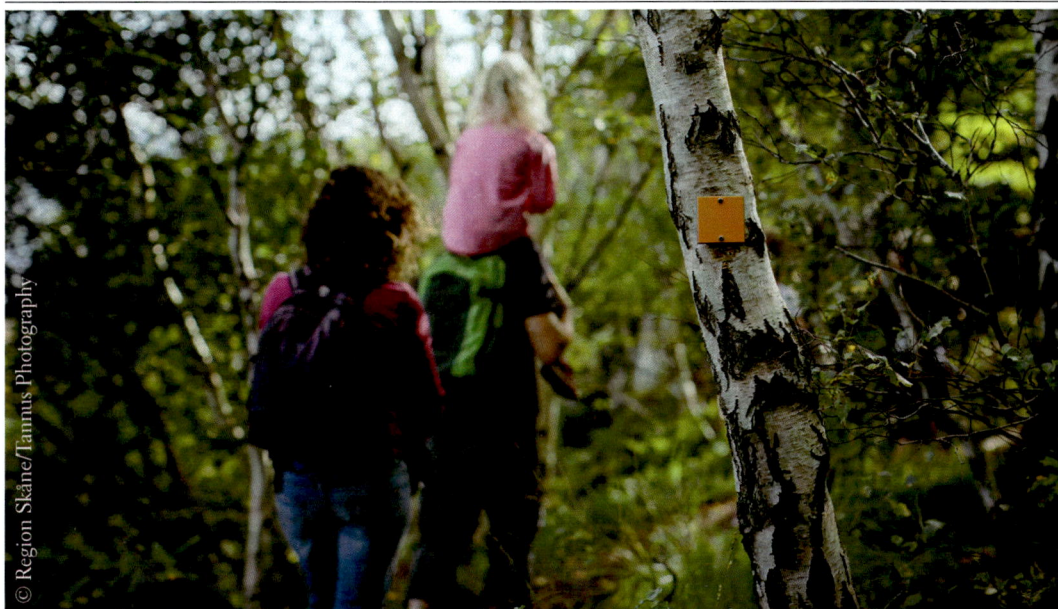

Region Skåne's public health and social sustainability goals

Against the background of Health 2020, the national public health policy goals and the regional development strategy, Region Skåne's public health work has three goals:

1. good health and life quality for all citizens of Skåne
2. more equal and socially sustainable community development
3. a good start in life for children and young people from a life-course perspective (26).

Implementation – moving from what to how

The action plan recognizes several existing strategies and policies across different units in Region Skåne that are linked to public health work. An important task for the action plan is, therefore, to clearly coordinate these strategies by developing intersectoral activities within the Public Health and Social Sustainability Unit's prioritized areas. With special focus on the social determinants for health, certain areas were prioritized to increase social sustainability in Skåne. These areas are connected to the relevant goals in *The open Skåne 2030 (3)* (Table 2).

A public health team is working to stimulate engagement and interest across the different sectors in Region Skåne and find its natural partners. The purpose is to find common and shared goals and indicators with other units, and then jointly identify ways for collaboration and activities for working across units.

Table 2. Goal indictors of public health and social sustainability

Priority areas	The open Skåne 2030 goal indicators
Public health reporting and systematic work with population surveillance data	• The health of the population shall have improved compared to 2014 and the differences shall have decreased as regards equality. • The share of Skåne's residents with good self-assessed health shall have increased compared to 2014, and the level shall be above the national average for all population groups and ages. • Child and youth self-assessed health shall have improved compared to 2014, and the share who are optimistic about the future shall have increased.
Employment and skills for growth and health	• The employment rate in Skåne shall be higher than the national average and reflect Skåne's population demographic. • Unemployment in Skåne shall be lower than the national average. • At least 85% of all 20-year-olds in Skåne shall have completed secondary school. • All students shall be eligible for tertiary education when finishing compulsory school at age 16.

Priority areas	The open Skåne 2030 goal indicators
Diversity, growth and health	• The citizenry's faith and participation in democracy shall be higher than in 2014. • The employment rate in Skåne shall be higher than the national average and reflect Skåne's population demographic. • The health of the population shall have improved compared to 2014, and the differences shall have decreased as regards equality.
Culture and health	• Everyone shall have the opportunity to participate in Skåne's cultural life and cultural experiences. • The share of Skåne's residents with good self-assessed health shall have increased compared to 2014, and the level shall be above the national average for all population groups and ages. • Skåne's residents shall be offered welfare services, including nurseries, schools, and health services or care services that are experienced as better and as higher quality than the national average.
Participation and influence	• The citizenry's faith and participation in democracy shall be higher than in 2014. • The health of the population shall have improved compared to 2014, and the differences shall have decreased as regards equality. • Skåne's residents shall be offered welfare services, including nurseries, schools, and health services or care services that are experienced as better and as higher quality than the national average.
Social sustainability in physical planning	• The health of the population shall have improved compared to 2014, and the differences shall have decreased as regards equality. • The employment rate in Skåne shall be higher than the national average and reflect Skåne's population demographic. • Accessibility shall have been improved such that Skåne's inhabitants can reach 80% of workplaces within 45 minutes using public transport. • 6000 homes shall have been constructed each year, with a diverse composition as regards rented/owned properties, size and building type, matching an annual population growth of 1%.

Table 2 contd

Priority areas	The open Skåne 2030 goal indicators
Environment and health	• The health of the population shall have improved compared to 2014 and the differences shall have decreased as regards equality. • Skåne shall have reached the environmental goals for the country. • Skåne shall be climate-neutral and fossil fuel-free. • The share of Skåne's residents with good self-assessed health shall have increased compared to 2014 and the level shall be above the national average for all population groups and ages. • Child and youth self-assessed health shall have improved compared to 2014 and the share who are optimistic about the future shall have increased.
Health promotion in health care	• The average life expectancy in Skåne shall be higher than the national average. • The health of the population shall have improved compared to 2014, and the differences shall have decreased as regards equality. • Child and youth self-assessed health shall have improved compared to 2014, and the share who are optimistic about the future shall have increased. • The share of Skåne's residents with good self-assessed health shall have increased compared to 2014 and the level shall be above the national average for all population groups and ages.

Sources: *The open Skåne 2030* (3); *A socially sustainable Skåne 2030. The action plan for Region Skåne's public health work 2015–2018* (26).

EVALUATION

An important part of the work with the regional development strategy is the follow-up of goals and indicators. The follow-up instrument *How has it gone in Skåne?* (27) provides indicators for all the target goals in *The open Skåne 2030* (3). *How has it gone in Skåne?* is compiled annually to follow up how Skåne has developed with regards to a number of chosen indicators. A website (25) has statistics and tables that can be tailored for specific needs (27).

Fifteen of the nearly 30 goal indicators in *The open Skåne 2030* measure health and the social determinants of health (Table 2).

Data are collected from sources including Statistics Sweden, which is responsible for supporting and coordinating the Swedish system for official statistics, and Region Skåne's public health surveys that carry out epidemiological monitoring and surveillance in the entire population of Skåne. These enable links to be made between the social determinants of health and health equity outcomes in order to support the county and municipalities at local level with their health planning and decision-making.

Fig. 3–4 illustrate the findings of one of the public health surveys. This shows the socioeconomic differences in health, lifestyles and living conditions among men and women compared to a reference group of white-collar workers (28).

Fig. 3. Socioeconomic status of men aged 18–64 years in Skåne

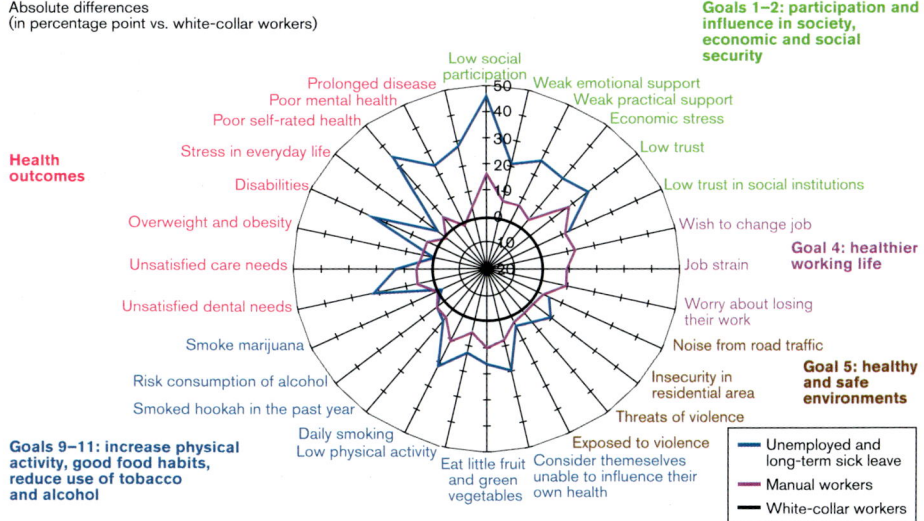

Source: adapted and reproduced by permission from Region Skåne (28).

Implementation – moving from what to how

Fig. 4. Socioeconomic status of women aged 18–64 years in Skåne

Absolute differences
(in percentage point vs. white-collar workers)

Health outcomes
- Prolonged disease
- Poor mental health
- Poor self-rated health
- Stress in everyday life
- Disabilities
- Overweight and obesity
- Unsatisfied care needs
- Unsatisfied dental needs
- Smoke marijuana
- Risk consumption of alcohol
- Smoked hookah in the past year
- Daily smoking
- Low physical activity
- Eat little fruit and green vegetables

Goals 9–11: increase physical activity, good food habits, reduce use of tobacco and alcohol

Goals 1–2: participation and influence in society, economic and social security
- Low social participation
- Weak emotional support
- Weak practical support
- Economic stress
- Low trust
- Low trust in social institutions

Goal 4: healthier working life
- Wish to change job
- Job strain
- Worry about losing their work

Goal 5: healthy and safe environments
- Noise from road traffic
- Insecurity in residential area
- Threats of violence
- Exposed to violence
- Consider themselves unable to influence their own health

— Unemployed and long-term sick leave
— Manual workers
— White-collar workers

Source: adapted and reproduced by permission from Region Skåne (28).

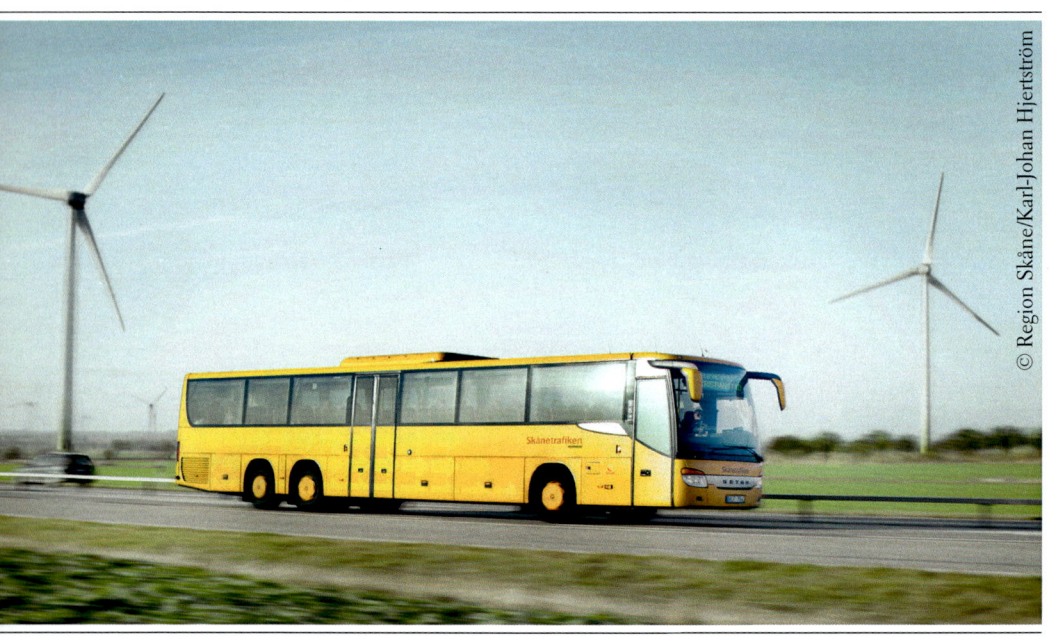

© Region Skåne/Karl-Johan Hjertström

Challenges and strengths of the process

CHALLENGES

Find the common voice and emphasize the whole. A key challenge was how to create one voice among all the municipalities, as gains by one municipality was seen as a loss for another. Through continued and regular dialogue, Region Skåne's approach was to emphasis the potential for Skåne when speaking with one common voice in the national arena. The message was that every municipality was important to the coherent whole. Citizens also do not see the boundaries of a municipality, but rather want to have one functioning labour market and be able to move freely throughout the whole of Skåne.

Work towards the common and issue-driven good. With five significant cities, Skåne is, in principle, divided into two labour market regions: Malmö/Lund/Helsingborg and Hässelholm/Kristianstad. It is an unusual example of a multinuclear, polycentric local structure and has the highest density area in Sweden. This brings benefits as inhabitants are in close proximity to cities, smaller towns, forests, the sea, work and various types of living. It also poses challenges in terms of a functioning infrastructure, how to take advantage of internal differences and how to develop the interaction between the major strategic actors within Skåne. This demands an ability to manage multilevel steering, **take a whole-of-government approach** and to develop a common regional identity. Again, it is about enabling municipalities to see beyond their own boundaries, and work for a common and issue-driven good. For example, where one municipality's strength is to offer accommodation, another might offer a plurality of works and education. Together, they represent an attractive whole for those who live and work in Skåne. Furthermore, a polycentric regional structure offers a sustainable approach for controlling the growth of urbanization.

Think in terms of one's organization, as well as a wider region. The ultimate ambition of the regional strategy is to bring about change in what the citizens think about Skåne, so they feel that Skåne is a functional and attractive region. To achieve this, people who are working locally need to think not only about their own organization, but also in terms of what is best for their region. To do this, they need to encapsulate the regional strategy within their core values and ground it in their daily work activities. Measuring and articulating this impact over time is challenging. Region Skåne is presently assessing how to achieve this.

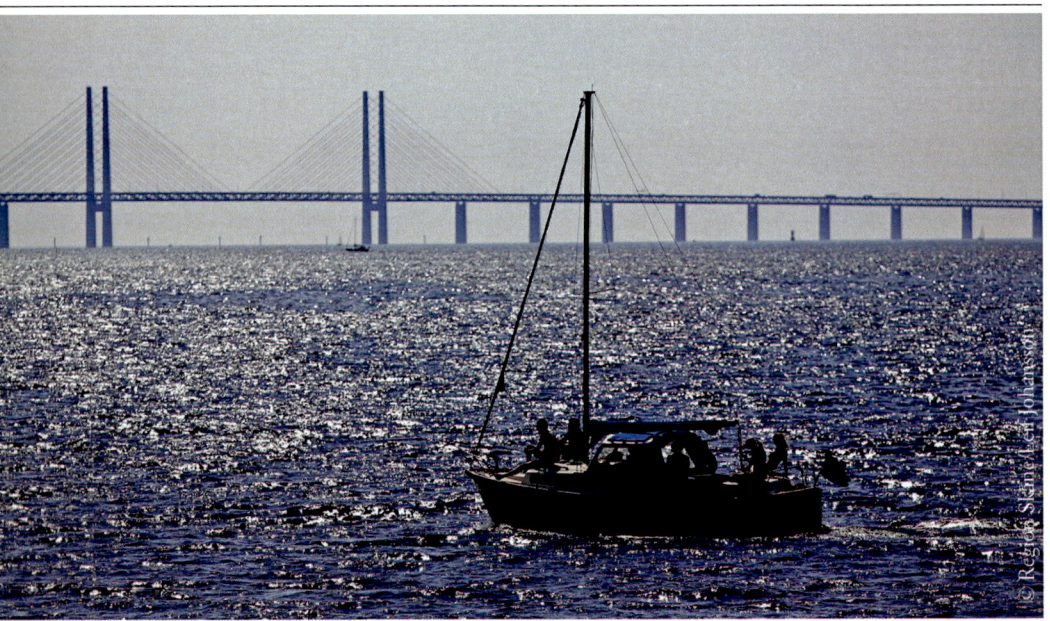

Strengths

Be mindful about leadership roles. A success factor in the work with the regional development strategy was the Chair of the Political Steering Group, a senior-level politician with many years' experience in regional development. This enabled her to maturely tackle the broad scope of work that newer politicians would have found overwhelming, and use her political standing and connections.

Engage in a longer-term plan that considers champions for implementation. For continued success, a decisive factor is the new politicians both in Region Skåne and the municipalities. They have ownership of the vision of open Skåne 2030 and think it is particularly important to steer their respective activities towards the common goals. For this to be possible requires more in-depth dialogues to discuss the regional development strategy from the viewpoint of a region, and the municipality's specific opportunities and challenges. A common thread is needed, from the development strategy to the daily work activities, so professionals can feel the relevance and understand how to drive it forward and create a feeling that together they can realize open Skåne 2030.

Involve networks that can support the process. Skåne's Leaders Forum, though a relatively new arena for the open Skåne, has been significant in maintaining momentum for the regional development work. This network comprises leaders from Region Skåne, the County Administrative Board of Skåne and the Swedish Association of Local Authorities and Regions who meet to discuss issues of strategic importance for development in Skåne, and how to create conditions for a collected regional behaviour.

A trustworthy brand has merit. A large enabling factor was the Region Skåne brand. Since its establishment in 1999, it has built itself up to be a trustworthy brand. In addition, it has the power that comes with the responsibility of managing budgets derived mainly from local taxes. Coupled with this, it had the maturity to take a unified approach with municipalities rather than rely on its authority from the State's mandate to coordinate the regional development work. The honesty put forth about the challenges faced by Skåne was seen as refreshing especially from a political perspective.

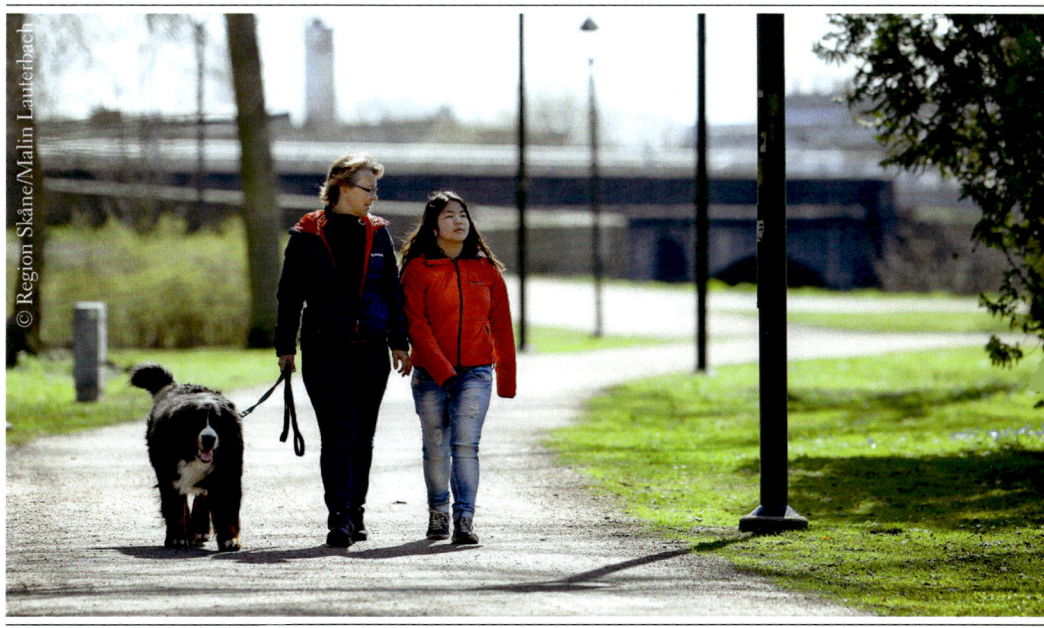

Joint action for development

> *Realising a joint strategy requires time, humility and trust. Creating the open Skåne requires cooperation, in which several actors and individual people act on a certain challenge at the right time. Acting alone is not conducive to the transition to a sustainable society (3).*

Joint mobilization requires special abilities and expertise. An important ability is to identify which challenges or opportunities require joint action. Another is to be able to gather actors on cross-sector platforms, so that a broad approach can be used. It requires leadership characterized by courage, a willingness to take risks and, at the same time, an openness to invite all stakeholder views and initiatives, in order to challenge prevailing ideas and adapt to new circumstances.

The journey towards the open Skåne is not one process with one given leader. Rather, it involves different actors from state to local level and across all sectors that will lead from time to time. The work is based on feedback and continual dialogue, into which new knowledge and new perspectives are continually infused. It also requires that different actors shoulder responsibility for their areas of expertise and the involvement of citizenry.

Strong joint actions do not negate the fact that 33 municipalities continue to work and develop individually. The power to act for Skåne's development emerges from a dialogue between the local and regional levels, with a basis in their different circumstances. This also applies to companies, associations and other types of organizations.

The benefits of cooperating and highlighting each other's strengths are many. Allowing the most suitable actor to lead at the right time shortens lead times, and everyone learns from each other. Moreover, engaging the right actor at the right time in the process creates a clear driving force that provides a clear direction. Cooperation entails not to compromise, but rather to complement and strengthen one another. This is not always a straightforward process; naturally, some actors are more sceptical about coordination, and building trust between stakeholders takes time. Work like this is about give and take, so satisfying everyone all the time is not possible.

By actively working in multiple stages so as to include multiple actors and to gather input from ongoing initiatives, Skåne's regional development strategy has taken shape (Fig. 5). This must hold true when the actors take joint action to develop the open Skåne. The work with the development strategy entails creating a common foundation, as well as joint commitment to and shared responsibility for Skåne's development.

Fig. 5. Reciprocal joint action

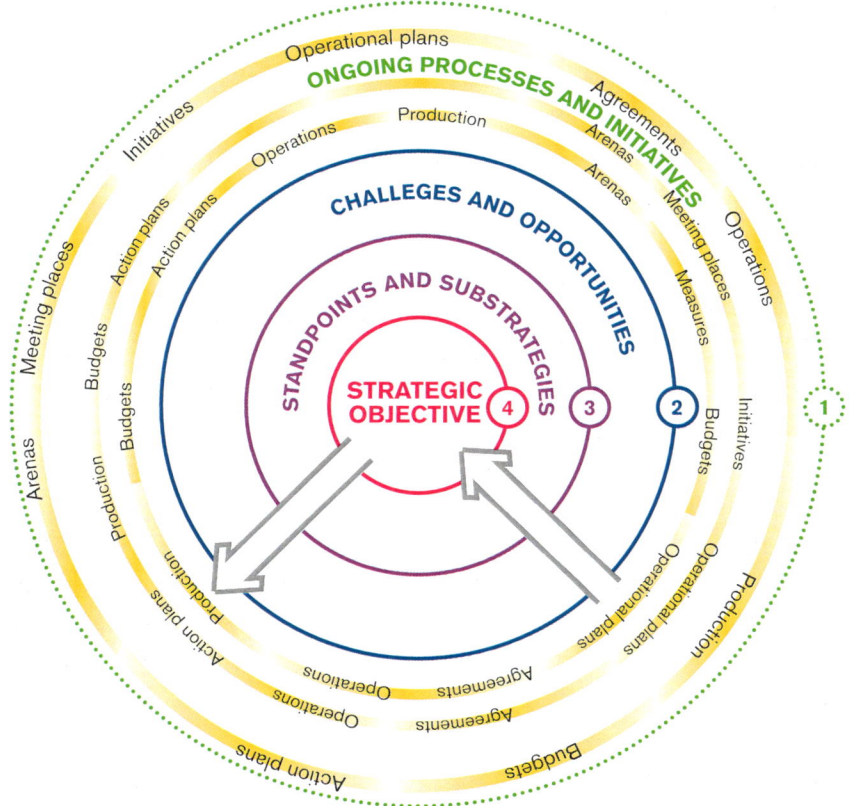

Source: reproduced with permission from Region Skåne (3).

In the various ongoing parallel processes, one or more actors identifies an opportunity, takes a joint stance and formulates a joint strategic objective, which is what Region Skåne wanted to achieve.

Based on the jointly processed strategic objective, priorities and standpoints are made that fulfil the different opportunities and challenges, which result in different processes and actors being activated, which in turn results in initiatives and actions.

Skåne's development entails actors and processes moving around continually in this mutual interaction. These movements create new conditions and opportunities, new ideas and collaborations – new movement – the ecosystem in motion.

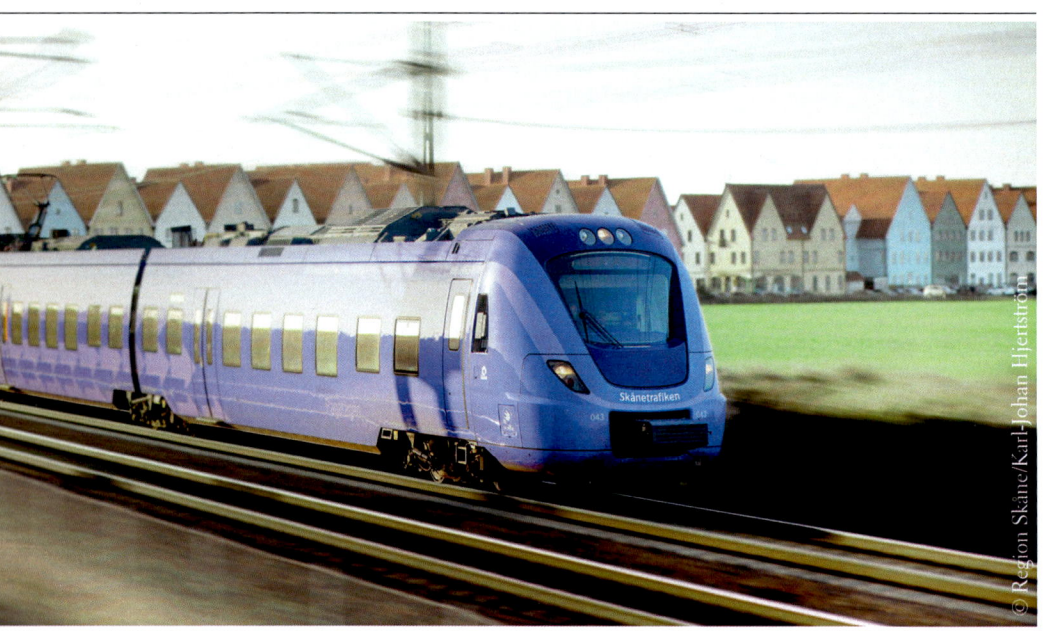

Key messages

Find a common purpose for stakeholders. Emphasize the potential of the common good or the common issue when working as a connected whole, and enable people to see beyond their boundaries.

Focus on the process rather than the product. Creating ownership and involvement from all stakeholders is much harder than producing a policy product. Identify the common driving force as to why everyone is doing this, and determine the new behaviour and norms everyone wants.

Trust the process. Be a sounding board that moves in between stakeholders like a free agent (or a broker or convener), and guide the process by being receptive and flowing with rather than controlling it. Trust that stakeholders will jointly make the best informed decisions for a region.

Emphasize governance processes involving people and power over constructing a formal framework of structures. Winning people's hearts through building trust and by giving them more responsibility is essential. Human and social capital are also essential, and hence necessary to provide skills on how to be a free agent (or broker or convener). Providing skills development can support the growth of individual and organizational competencies.

Create ownership of the process through leadership and ambassadors, and engagement with networks and alliances that will ultimately drive the process and maintain its momentum.

Involve and empower other sectors (not only health) by engaging the whole of the public sector, as well as communities and industries to share purpose, objectives and benefits.

Joint mobilization requires leadership characterized by courage, a willingness to take risks and, at the same time, an openness to invite all stakeholder views and initiatives in order to challenge prevailing ideas and adapt to new circumstances.

Do a background analysis first in order to assess the characteristics of the situation and the relevant stakeholders, so they can become involved as early as possible. Using a known independent body to give weight to the findings is useful.

Case studies

Autonomous Province of Trento (Italy)

This case study describes the shifting focus from health services to health promotion and from an expert-driven to a more participatory approach in the development of a health plan.

Background

The Autonomous Province of Trento is located in the northern part of Italy and has about 500 000 inhabitants. The National Health Service provides health services organized in a single local health unit (LHU) divided into four smaller health districts and 16 valley communities. A number of health surveillance systems (on behavioural risk factors of children, adults and the elderly) and other health-related data sources (such as mortality and cancer registry, hospital and emergency room discharge data) are available in this region.

The local health authority periodically assigns specific objectives and goals to the LHU on an annual basis, but, besides this, no comprehensive strategic health plan has been developed in the last 20 years. The annual epidemiological reports have been rich in data describing issues related to services provided by the LHU, but have given little information on population health, social determinants and the distribution of risk factors and resources in the community. Furthermore, health planning has not usually been based on systematic epidemiological data analysis but mostly on expert opinion.

What was needed

Firstly, the Health Observatory, Department of Health and Social Solidarity of the Autonomous Province of Trento wanted to draw attention to the determinants of health, in order to highlight the importance of health promotion and to support a shift to the health-in-all-policies approach in regional health planning. Another important issue was to enhance capacity building among health and social workers in connecting epidemiological analysis, prioritization, community participation and public health planning. The main goal remained to draft a strategic health plan taking into account WHO's Health 2020 (2) and health in all policies, and ensure the adoption of a participatory approach.

What was done

In 2012, the structure of the health report (29) and subsequent updates (30) were radically changed with paramount importance given to social determinants and population health conditions and risk factors. Consequently the former health services status report was replaced by a population health profile.

In 2013, with the help of the WHO Regional Office for Europe and the Regions for Health Network, the Health Observatory organized a training course on public health planning for key decision-makers both at the regional and health district levels.

In 2014, the Health Observatory set up a working group to develop the regional health plan with participation from both the health and social sectors. This group produced the first draft of the strategic health plan 2015–2025. The two main strategic objectives are:

- improving health for all and reducing health inequities
- improving governance for health.

These were broken down into three main goals:

- more years of healthy life for everyone (improving well-being and tackling the main health problems applying a life-course approach);
- health-promoting living and working conditions; and
- a person-centred health and social welfare system.

Finally, two overarching goals were added: reduction of health inequalities and improvement of health literacy.

At the end of 2014, a health-in-all-policies commission was set up involving all sectors of the regional government (such as environment, economy and transport). The commission drafted an inventory of health-related policies and programmes that would be integrated into the health plan.

Participatory approach

Between 2014 and 2015, institutional and social stakeholders were identified and a web-based platform *(31)* was developed to allow commentary on the draft health plan and the submission of new proposals.

In addition, the Health Observatory organized face-to-face meetings and workshops for stakeholders, and held onsite evening meetings with the health councils of all 16 local valley communities. In the first wave of the participatory approach, the platform was visited by 1926 users, and 210 opinions and evaluations were given; 60 new proposals were made and 21 documents with comments and proposals from a total of over 80 associations, NGOs and professional organizations were posted on the platform *(31)*.

Based on the comments and proposals, the draft was re-written: 41 out of 60 new proposals and around 60% of comments were summarized and integrated into the second version. A working group excluded comments considered too specific or too generic or that affirmed existing proposals or lacked feasibility. Overall, the second draft increased from 29 to 44 pages, and 14 new topics were added.

The second draft was open for discussion, comments and new proposals from the general public (April–June 2015), using the internet platform and meetings with the 16 valley communities.

In order to collect feedback and promote the use of the platform among members of the community, local facilitators were trained to identify local leaders representing different stakeholders in the community, and to organize local meetings and activities. This organization of local activities to promote participation was coordinated centrally, but how this was done was left to the valley communities to decide. Some used open space technology, and others used traditional community meetings or even excursions in the mountains with question and answer sessions.

In addition, the Health Observatory issued press releases, distributed postcards and bookmarks about how to participate, posted links to the internet platform on other websites (schools, LHU, immigration office, municipalities), and posted interviews about the health plan on YouTube. The Health Observatory created a newsletter and a website describing the planned activities and reported periodically about the planning process (32).

In the second wave of the participatory approach, between April and June 2015, the platform was visited by nearly 3000 users; 230 have been active users, mainly ordinary citizens of all ages, but also associations, NGOs, interest groups, school classes, community networks, etc. who posted a total of 690 comments and 140 new proposals.

Adding these numbers to those of the first wave (in which only health professionals and institutions were targeted), more than 1000 contributions (comments, ratings and new proposals) to the health plan have been made. At present, the working group of the Department of Health and Social Solidarity is writing the third draft of the health plan, which will take into account the proposals and comments of the second participatory wave.

Challenges

Despite strong and positive political commitment, at the beginning of the process, not everybody in the health and social service workforce really believed this participatory approach could work and some remain sceptical.

Political crisis and discussions about the re-organization of particular health services has captivated much of the public and professional attention on health-related issues hampering long-term reflection on health promotion.

The process conflicted with several regional laws regulating the establishment of separate health and social plans. Much time and energy was dedicated to writing a new law legalizing the process, and achieving the legal basis for a unified health and social plan.

Communication between different sectors and also among colleagues of the same sector but in different units was difficult, for example, because of personal issues and bureaucratic concerns about autonomy.

The draft had to be sound and well written but, at the same time, avoid giving the impression of a final document that would prevent participation.

The health plan had to be strategic, and contain pragmatic objectives and programmes that can be monitored and evaluated, rather than being too theoretical.

Some professional organizations and interest groups have used the participatory process to push their own agendas and specific projects.

Achieving the participation of the community (and health professionals) was difficult, because of lack of confidence in the authenticity and effectiveness of the process. This combined with a certain amount of passivity among the population who, if at all, were interested in the solution of short-term organizational problems of the health system but not in strategic planning for health promotion.

Next steps

The Health Observatory will hold a series of scientific seminars on a selection of topics included in the health plan. Based on the results of the second round of participation, a final version of the health plan will be drafted and presented to the Government for approval, hopefully by autumn 2015.

Autonomous Community of Andalusia (Spain)

This case study describes the experience of a participatory approach in designing, implementing and assessing the Fourth Andalusian Health Plan (IV AHP) (33).

Background

IV AHP, approved in December 2013, is the driver of most of the health plans, programmes and activities at regional, provincial and local levels in the Autonomous Community of Andalusia, the biggest autonomous region

(8 392 635 inhabitants) of Spain. By aiming to protect and improve the health status of the Andalusian population by addressing the determinants and living conditions that affect them, involving all policies in the process, IV AHP grounds its principles in Health 2020 (2).

In accordance with the whole-of-society approach suggested by Health 2020, participation was conceived as a key feature of IV AHP from the start. Promoting citizen participation in health-related issues is a cornerstone of IV AHP, as a way for developing the right to participate in public health policies as stated in the Public Health Act of Andalusia, Law 16/2011 (34). Participation is considered an asset for health, and a tool for democratic development and improving health care quality. The identification, monitoring and evaluation of tools and procedures for citizen participation in health policies can be considered one of the important tasks in the process of implementing IV AHP.

Process

Participation was included from the very beginning when the evaluation of the previous AHP (III AHP) was carried out. Citizens associations, patient associations and professionals participated.

Members of academia, health sector professionals and other government sectors in charge of policies affecting the social determinants of health were invited and participated in working groups to generate proposals for the new health plan.

Citizens associations, patient associations and professional unions and associations were involved in informing the technical proposal produced by working groups.

Finally, an official public hearing process was open to all citizens and associations before the official approval of IV AHP.

Summary

In total, 28 social and administrative authorities participated in the working groups during the development of IV AHP; 77 representatives of social and administrative actors and authorities were invited to the participation workshop to consider the technical proposal produced by working groups. Finally, 33 bodies and organizations submitted formal statements during the official public hearing process launched before the approval.

The participation of non-health government sectors (regional ministries), in line with health-in-all-policies and the whole-of-government approaches, was carried out through specific actions oriented towards the achievement of the main aims of IV AHP. Each sector identified actions within its own policies that could contribute to achieving the commitments of IV AHP. A description of actions, including the responsible sector, the allocated budget, the assessment procedure and the list of other involved sectors, was elaborated and contracted between the health government sectors and the other sectors.

A participatory process is currently being implemented at provincial and local levels, in the eight provinces and 774 municipalities of the Autonomous Community of Andalusia. The objective is to assess and rank the provincial and local health needs through a combination of participation forums, face-to-face discussion forums, a citizen's panel and panels of experts to produce a technical proposal for each provincial health plan. A so-called provincial day with associations that will consider and discuss the technical proposal and the official public hearing process ends this participatory process at the provincial level.

The definition of the health profile, the process of ranking the health needs and their resulting actions plans have been developed through municipal citizen and expert groups in more than 100 municipalities to date.

The spirit of IV AHP includes participation in the periodical and final evaluations, and is stated in the evaluation section of the III AHP.

Challenges

One of the most difficult steps in this process was related to the participation of the formal representatives of other regional ministry sectors. During the drafting of the AHP, two regional government changes took place, affecting those involved in the negotiation process. Each new regional ministry team, therefore, needed to start from the beginning and explain the health in all policies strategy, and the relevance of the impact of their policies on the health of the population and on their determinants.

Other challenges were the:

- differences in participation at regional, provincial and local levels;
- diversity of a participative culture in sectors other than health;
- need for participative procedures tending to promote a more bottom-up participative approach;
- need and opportunity for all sectors and participants to learn how to develop a more effective participative culture in designing policies;
- need to develop approaches for true participation of those with more needs; and
- implementation of an equity perspective in the participation process.

Wales (United Kingdom)

This case study illustrates participatory approaches to improving health and well-being in Wales for the present and future generations.

Background

Wales is one of the four United Kingdom nations with devolved powers (autonomy) in areas including health, housing, local government, environment, transport, education and culture (35). Overall, the health of the Welsh population is improving but inequalities remain a serious problem, similar to the rest of the United Kingdom and other regions in Europe (36).

Formal and informal recognition that public services have a central role in supporting individuals to maintain and improve their health and well-being is increasing. This requires public bodies to have greater engagement with individuals and communities. One example of emerging participatory mechanisms for health is co-production, which involves the sharing of power between professionals and citizens, enabling an equal partnership based on reciprocity; developing peer networks to give people a voice; and achieving outcomes that matter to individuals (37). Through such participatory approaches, the Well-being of Future Generations (Wales) Act 2015 (38) has been introduced that commits public bodies across Wales to improving the well-being of its citizens while taking the needs of future generations into account.

The Act provides a timely opportunity to shape the future of public services in the context of the forthcoming Sustainable Development Goals (39). It strengthens national commitment to sustainable development – the "process of improving the economic, social, environmental and cultural well-being of Wales" (38). The Act is both a key achievement in itself and a unique opportunity for establishing a truly participatory approach in Wales. It represents a milestone, recognizing and focusing on well-being (and health as part of it) as an element of and prerequisite for sustainable development.

Participatory approach

A highly participatory approach informed the Act, including a national conversation where the Welsh Government invited members of the public to express their aspirations for *The Wales we want report* (40). This involved over 7000 people across the country through public meetings with communities/groups and individual communications via social media, postcards or online. The Welsh Government recruited so-called future champions to act as advocates for future generations and raise issues that affect their communities or organizations. The national conversation has been augmented by a series of stakeholder workshops involving public service organizations. "The Wales we want" has mirrored the United Nations conversation on "The world we want" to support citizen participation in defining a new global development framework. It is intended that the development of local plans and statutory guidance will follow a similar process building on the sustainable development expertise across Wales. In addition, the legislative process by which the Act received Royal Assent involved a participatory approach, whereby interested stakeholders provided written and oral evidence during the scrutiny process.

Enabling participation through the Act

The participatory approach to well-being is now a legal duty and responsibility. Enforced from April 2016, all public bodies will share responsibility for achieving seven statutory well-being goals.

- A prosperous Wales is an innovative, productive, low-carbon economy, generating wealth and employment for a skilled and well-educated population.
- A resilient Wales is a biodiverse environment with healthy functioning ecosystems that support social, economic and ecological resilience.
- A healthier Wales is a society in which physical and mental well-being is maximized and in which choices and behaviours that benefit health are understood.
- A more equal Wales is a society that enables people to fulfil their potential, regardless of background or circumstances.
- A Wales of cohesive communities is attractive, viable, safe and well-connected.
- A Wales of vibrant culture and thriving Welsh language is a society that promotes and protects culture and heritage, encouraging participation in the arts and sport.
- A globally responsible Wales is a nation which, when doing anything to improve well-being in Wales, takes into account making a positive contribution to global well-being (38).

Public bodies will be required to set and accomplish well-being objectives that will maximize their contribution to achieving well-being goals. Public bodies will need to work jointly through public services boards (PSBs), established for each local authority area in Wales. PSBs will consist of statutory members e.g. the local authority, the local health board, the fire and rescue authority and Natural Resources Wales, as well as invited participants e.g. local county voluntary councils and other partners, for example, community councils. PSBs are required to publish a well-being assessment to inform the development of a local well-being plan, maximizing their contribution to the achievement of the Act goals. National indicators will be published to measure collective progress. The Act also makes provision to establish the Future Generations Commissioner to advise, support, monitor and review public bodies. A new duty has been placed on the Auditor General for Wales to assess how public bodies have applied the sustainable development principle, including the well-being objectives.

Involving citizens and communities is embedded within various aspects of the Act. For example, public bodies are required to act 'in accordance with the sustainable development principle' by taking account of five areas: involvement, long-term thinking, integration, collaboration and prevention *(38)*. Here involvement means involving people and communities with an interest in the well-being goals, and collaboration means public bodies having a shared responsibility for contributing to well-being goals.

The Act is an important opportunity to further develop a **health-in-all-policies approach**. To achieve this, Public Health Wales has called for the inclusion of a health impact assessment process in all policy developments and decisions. The purpose is to enable the wider determinants of health to be viewed through a so-called health lens and to provide opportunities to engage with local communities. In addition, Public Health Wales is publishing a health in all policies guidance, adapting and applying the theory and evidence to the Welsh context.

Early **feedback from** local authorities who are part of a Future Generations **Early Adopters** scheme indicate positive outcomes in respect of improving health and well-being. For example, in Swansea, the health impact assessment has been integrated into the local land use development planning and associated developments.

In conclusion

Legislation is arguably one of the most powerful tools available to governments to direct long-term policy goals for health and well-being, and to lever positive changes in society. The principles of community participation and involvement have become fundamental for good public health policy and practice globally, as well as in Wales *(41)*.

The Act, developed through a conversation with Welsh citizens, is consistent with international ambitions to set goals that link population well-being with consideration of future generations. The Act provides a sustainable national plan and places Wales in a position to engage with the United Nations Sustainable Development Goals (39).

References[1]

1. Review of social determinants and the health divide in the WHO European Region. Final report. Copenhagen: WHO Regional Office for Europe; 2013 (http://www.euro.who.int/en/health-topics/health-policy/health-2020-the-european-policy-for-health-and-well-being/the-evidence/review-of-social-determinants-and-the-health-divide-in-the-who-european-region.-final-report).

2. Health 2020. A European policy framework and strategy for the 21st century. Copenhagen: WHO Regional Office for Europe; 2013 (http://www.euro.who.int/en/health-topics/health-policy/health-2020-the-european-policy-for-health-and-well-being/publications/2013/health-2020-a-european-policy-framework-and-strategy-for-the-21st-century).

3. The open Skåne 2030. Skåne's regional development strategy June 2014. Kristianstad: Region Skåne; 2014 (http://skane2030.se/det-oppna-skane/#prettyPhoto/1/).

4. European Union Strategy for the Baltic Sea Region [website]. Brussels: European Commission; 2015 (http://www.balticsea-region-strategy.eu/).

5. Europe 2020. A strategy for smart, sustainable and inclusive growth. Brussels: European Commission; 2010 (http://eur-lex.europa.eu/LexUriServ/LexUriServ.do?uri=COM:2010:2020:FIN:EN:PDF).

6. 2030 framework for climate and energy policies. In: European Commission [website]. Brussels: European Commission; 2015 (http://ec.europa.eu/clima/policies/2030/index_en.htm).

7. Cohesion policy frequently asked questions. In: European Commission [website]. Brussels: European Commission; 2015 (http://ec.europa.eu/regional_policy/en/faq/).

8. An international innovation strategy for Skåne 2012–2020. Kristianstad: Skåne Research and Innovation Council, Sounding Board for Innovation in Skåne; 2011 (https://www.skane.se/Upload/Webbplatser/Naringsliv/Dokument/IIFS%20Strategi%20Version%20Slutligt%20dokument%20Orginal%20Version%202012-2020.pdf).

9. Strategies for the polycentric Skåne. Kristianstad: Region Skåne, Department for Planning and Urban Development; 2013 (http://utveckling.skane.se/publikationer/strategier-och-planer/strategies-for-the-polycentric-skane/).

---

[1] Online resources were accessed on 7 August 2015.

10. Göteborg Manifesto. Copenhagen: WHO Regional Office for Europe; 2012 (http://www.euro.who.int/en/about-us/networks/regions-for-health-network-rhn/publications/2012/the-regions-for-health-network-goteborg-manifesto).

11. Health and sustainable development. Key health trends. Geneva: World Health Organization; 2002 (http://www.who.int/mediacentre/events/HSD_Plaq_02.2_Gb_def1.pdf?ua=1).

12. United Nations World Commission on Environment and Development. Report of the World Commission on Environment and Development: our common future. Oxford: Oxford University Press; 1987 (http://www.un-documents.net/wced-ocf.htm).

13. Preamble to the Constitution of the World Health Organization as adopted by the International Health Conference, New York, 19–22 June 1946; signed on 22 July 1946 by the representatives of 61 States (Official Records of the World Health Organization, no. 2, p. 100) and entered into force on 7 April 1948 (http://www.who.int/about/definition/en/print.html).

14. What is participatory health research? Version: May 2013. Berlin: International Collaboration for Participatory Health Research; 2013 (Position paper 1; http://www.icphr.org/uploads/2/0/3/9/20399575/ichpr_position_paper_1_defintion_-_version_may_2013.pdf).

15. Winter R. Truth or fiction: problems of validity and authenticity in narratives of action research. Educational Action Research. 2002;10(1):143–54.

16. McNiff J. Action research: principles and practice, first edition. London: Routledge; 1992.

17. Statistics database. In: Statistics Sweden [website]. Stockholm: Statistics Sweden; 2015 (http://www.statistikdatabasen.scb.se/).

18. Skåne County – Facts and figures. In: Region facts [website]. Luleå: Pantzare Information; 2015 (http://www.regionfakta.com/Skane-lan/IN-ENGLISH/Geography-/).

19. Organisation for Economic Co-operation and Development. OECD territorial reviews: Skåne, Sweden 2012. Paris: OECD Publishing; 2012 (http://dx.doi.org/10.1787/9789264177741-en).

20. Organisation for Economic Co-operation and Development. OECD territorial reviews: Sweden 2010. Paris: OECD Publishing; 2010 (http://www.keepeek.com/Digital-Asset-Management/oecd/urban-rural-and-regional-development/oecd-territorial-reviews-sweden-2010_9789264081888-en).

21. Regional development programme for Skåne 2009–2016. Region Skåne; 2010 (https://www.skane.se/Public/Skaneportalen-extern/Skanes_utveckling/RUP_ENG_.pdf).

22. Örtengren K. The logical framework approach. A summary of the theory behind the LFA method. Stockholm: Swedish Agency for International Development Cooperation; 2003.

23. About the project ESS MAX IV in the region: TITA. In: Skåne [website]. Kristianstad: Region Skåne; 2015 (http://essmax4tita.skane.org/en/content/about-project).

24. Structural picture of Skåne – future challenges. Kristianstad: Region Skåne, Department of Regional Development; 2010 (http://utveckling.skane.se/siteassets/publikationer_dokument/strukturbild_future_challenges.pdf).

25. Det öppna Skåne 2030 [The open Skåne 2030] [website]. Kristianstad: Region Skåne; 2015 (http://skane2030.se/) (in Swedish).

26. Ett socialt hållbart Skåne 2030. Handlingsplan för Region Skånes folkhälsoarbete 2015–2018. [A socially sustainable Skåne 2030. The action plan for Region Skåne's public health work 2015–2018]. Kristianstad: Region Skåne, Public Health and Social Sustainability Unit; 2015 (http://utveckling.skane.se/siteassets/folkhalsa_och_social_hallbarht/dokument/handlingsplan-rs-folkhalsoarbete-slutversion.pdf) (in Swedish).

27. Hur har det gått i Skåne? 2014 års uppföljning av regionalt utvecklingsarbete. [How has it gone in Skåne? The 2014 evaluation of the regional development work]. Kristianstad: Region Skåne, Urban Planning Unit; 2014 (http://rapport.skane.se/huga/pdfs/Huga2014_hela_rapporten.pdf) (in Swedish).

28. Folkhälsorapport Skåne 2013: en undersökning om vuxnas livsvillkor, levnadsvanor och hälsa [The public health report Skåne 2013: a study about adult's living conditions, lifestyles and health]. Kristianstad: Region Skåne, Public Health and Social Sustainability Unit; 2013 (http://utveckling.skane.se/publikationer/rapporter-analyser-och-prognoser/folkhalsorapport-skane-2013/) (in Swedish).

29. Centre for Health of the Autonomous Province of Trento. Profilo di salute della provincia di Trento 2012 N. 9 [Health profile of the province of Trento 2012 no. 9]. Trento: Council of the Autonomous Province of Trento; 2012 (http://www.trentinosalute.net/Contenuti/Pubblicazioni/Focus/9-Profilo-di-salute-della-provincia-di-Trento-2012) (in Italian).

30. Centre for Health of the Autonomous Province of Trento, editors. Profilo di salute della provincia di Trento – Aggiornamento 2014 N. 14 [Health profile of the province of Trento – 2014 update no. 14]. Trento: Council of the Autonomous Province of Trento; 2014 (http://www.trentinosalute.net/Contenuti/Pubblicazioni/Focus/14-Profilo-di-salute-della-provincia-di-Trento-Aggiornamento-2014) (in Italian).

31. Verso il Piano per la salute del Trentino (2015–2025) [The plan for the health of Trentino (2015–2025)]. In: Autonomous Province of Trento [website]. Trento: Autonomous Province of Trento; 2015 (http://pianosalute.partecipa.tn.it) (in Italian).

32. Io racconto, storie di salute [I tell, stories of health]. In: Autonomous Province of Trento [website]. Trento: Autonomous Province of Trento; 2015 (https://ioracconto.partecipa.tn.it/story/ioracconto_storie_di_salute) (in Italian).

33. Fourth Andalusian Health Plan. Executive summary. Seville: Government of Andalusia Department of Equality, Health and Social Policy; 2013 (http://www.juntadeandalucia.es/salud/sites/csalud/galerias/documentos/c_1_c_6_planes_estrategias/IV_plan_andaluz_salud/IV_PAS_v9_english.pdf).

34. Article 15 of the Public Health Act of Andalusia, Law 16/2011 of 23 December 2011. Seville: Government of Andalusia; 2011.

35. Devolution Settlement: Wales, 20 February 2013. In: Government of the United Kingdom [website]. London: Government of the United Kingdom; 2015 (https://www.gov.uk/devolution-settlement-wales).

36. Welsh Health Survey. Release date 28 January 2015. In: Welsh Government [website]. Cardiff: Welsh Government; 2015 (http://gov.wales/statistics-and-research/welsh-health-survey/?lang=en).

37. Making prudent health care happen [website]. Cardiff: Welsh Government; 2015 (http://www.prudenthealth care.org.uk/).

38. Well-being of Future Generations (Wales) Act 2015. Cardiff: National Assembly for Wales; 2015 (http://www.legislation.gov.uk/anaw/2015/2/enacted).

39. Open working group proposal for sustainable development goals. New York: United Nations; 2014 (https://sustainabledevelopment.un.org/index.php?page=view&type=400&nr=1579&menu=1300).

40. Welsh Government. The Wales we want report. A report on behalf of future generations. Cardiff: Welsh Government; 2015 (http://thewaleswewant.co.uk/wales-we-want-report).

41. Declaration of Alma-Ata. Geneva: World Health Organization; 1978 (http://www.euro.who.int/en/publications/policy-documents/declaration-of-alma-ata,-1978).